Praise for *Asylum on the Hill*

"This well-written, accurately researched historical work tells the story of the Athens Lunatic Asylum. . . . This is a work that brings the reader inside the life and times of patient care in Ohio. *Asylum on the Hill* is highly readable, enlightening, and for those who currently work in the field of psychiatry, the story is familiar and somewhat poignant. . . . *Highly recommended.*"

—*Choice*

"*Asylum on The Hill* is a fascinating and poignant history of one hospital, its patients and staff. Accompanied by rare, never released photos and records, Ziff's easy narrative weaves the personal accounts of daily life with the broader context of post-Civil War America. What's truly remarkable about Ziff's book is that it tells a parallel story of our nation's history and the forces that shaped not only the asylums but also the many other fundamental public institutions that survive today. A highly engaging work that makes the past come alive."

—Christopher Payne, author of *Asylum: Inside the Closed World of State Mental Hospitals*

"Anyone who peruses Ziff's work will not have an easy time putting it down. This book is more than a history of a time, a place, a movement, and a people. It is instead a sensitive and centered examination. . . . Her portraits of people who influenced the asylum are wonderfully rendered . . . alive and moving."

—Samuel T. Gladding, Wake Forest University

"People interested in the history of Ohio University's Ridges property—and there are many such in this area—may think they've struck a gold mine if they open a new book issued by the OU Press."

—*Athens News*

"This is a study of the efforts, trials, and successes of the first twenty years of the Athens Lunatic Asylum under the rubric of the concept of moral treatment. Ziff's work is the first of its kind in looking at the earliest decades of this rural and cutting-edge asylum and she does a wonderful job of presenting the story in the broad context of the state of asylums in America as well as the specific context of this asylum in Athens, Ohio."

—Douglas McCabe,
retired curator of manuscripts, Ohio University

"By telling the story of one institution, Ziff places in context the larger picture of how professionals and the lay public thought about and cared for less fortunate individuals. Readers with diverse interests such as the history of psychiatry, medico-sociological analysis, and mid-to-late nineteenth-century politics will enjoy this book."

—*Metapsychology*

"Katherine Ziff's fascinating *Asylum on the Hill* concentrates on the first 20 years of the institution, from 1874 to 1893, when it was a cutting-edge example of progressive care for the mentally ill. . . . Ziff's detailed research into patient records and letters yields tantalizing glimpses into the lives of those taken into the asylum, as well as those of staff members. . . . The volume is amply illustrated with period photographs, reproductions of letters, maps, tables and postcards."

—*Columbus Dispatch*

"Ziff's narrative—skillfully interwoven with period photos and excerpts from letters and reports—keeps the reader firmly rooted in the benevolent mindset of the time. While also covering negative aspects such as endemic political patronage and eventual overcrowding, it is, nevertheless, a lovely glimpse at a kinder and gentler time in Ohio's treatment of its mentally ill."

—Thomas Walker, *Ohio Today*

"*Asylum on the Hill* provides a valuable contribution to nineteenth-century American history and to the history of medicine."

—*Indiana Magazine of History*

ASYLUM ON THE HILL

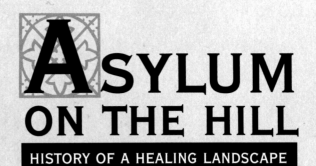

ASYLUM
ON THE HILL

HISTORY OF A HEALING LANDSCAPE

KATHERINE ZIFF

Foreword by Samuel T. Gladding

Afterword to the 150th Anniversary Edition by
Shawna Bolin and Joseph C. Shields

Ohio University Press Athens

Ohio University Press, Athens, Ohio 45701
ohioswallow.com
© 2012 by Ohio University Press
All rights reserved

First paperback edition printed in 2018
ISBN 978-0-8214-2341-7

Printed in the United States of America
Ohio University Press books are printed on acid-free paper ⊗ ™

HARDCOVER 25 24 23 22 21 20 19 18 17   7 6 5 4 3
PAPERBACK 26 25 24 23 22 21 20 19 18   5 4 3 2 1

Library of Congress Cataloging-in-Publication Data
Ziff, Katherine K.
 Asylum on the hill : history of a healing landscape / Katherine Ziff ; foreword
by Samuel T. Gladding.
    p. ; cm.
 Includes bibliographical references and index.
   ISBN 978-0-8214-1973-1 (hc : alk. paper)
 I. Title.
 [DNLM: 1. Athens Lunatic Asylum (Athens, Ohio) 2. Hospitals, Psychiatric
history Ohio. 3. Empathy Ohio. 4. History, 19th Century Ohio. 5. Mental
Disorders therapy Ohio. 6. Professional-Patient Relations Ohio. 7. Psychiatry
history Ohio.
 WM 28 AO3]

362.2109771 dc23

2011041136

Contents

FOREWORD

Some books are a joy to read. They are filled with information that is fascinating and informative. They entice you with their style, and before you know it you are into the text wholeheartedly and passionately. There is no logical explanation except that you are intrigued with what comes next and your expectations will not allow you to do anything else but read on. Katherine Ziff's *Asylum on the Hill: History of a Healing Landscape* is such a work. It covers a fascinating period in the history of American psychiatry that is now vanished but left an indelible mark for the positive and progressive impact it had on mental health care.

Dr. Ziff's focus on the Athens asylum is specific to the treatment of the mentally disturbed in Ohio in the late 1800s and captures a moment in time. It follows the ascendance of moral therapy as a movement that was humane and effective with those who were mentally distraught or thought to be such by their families and society. Ziff chronicles the lives of individuals who were admitted and treated, at least initially, from the moral therapy perspective. She humanizes notes made in the margins of official records of often-marginalized people who were in many ways similar to those with mental disorders today. Through a fascinating series of photographs, Dr. Ziff shows us what moral treatment was like in both the planning and the implementation of this unique way of helping the desperate, depressed, downtrodden, demented, anxious, and discouraged. She brings the reader into the sights, sounds, and even smells of post–Civil War America in Ohio. She describes, using the original records, the ways treatment for the "insane" worked and did not work—at least in this rural community in the Midwest.

Dr. Ziff gives us an insider's look at an asylum that dwarfed other buildings in its surroundings and, though carefully constructed, was not always lovingly cared for. She depicts the people—the patients and their families—who occupied the halls and challenged the minds of the times as individuals much like many Americans today. She traces the rationale for the moral therapy movement, its successes, and why it faded in its effectiveness and funding. She explains the reasons the movement, like those it touched, had a life but then failed to survive, let alone thrive. Her portraits of people who influenced the asylum are wonderfully rendered in words and pictures. This historical examination of the Hocking Valley, its people, and the asylum that impacted them is alive and moving. The extensive information within the pages of this text makes what was existentially enchanting relevant to our time.

Thus, when reading this book, a person is drawn past olden times and into scenes that have a universal dimension to them. The history of the past becomes a present reality; the people described become our neighbors—only from an earlier era. We can see ourselves and those we know in these individuals and in the treatment they received. Likewise, we know the caregivers, politicians, and landscapes within this story, for though shaped in the late 1800s, they are the forebearers and even the standard-bearers of the society that has since evolved and in which we live.

Anyone who peruses Ziff's work will not have an easy time putting it down. This book is more than a history of a time, a place, a movement, and a people. It is instead a sensitive and centered examination of growth and regression in the understanding of humankind amid stress, development, and regression. It is an exceptional peek into what life is and can be, along with what life has been. It is about a time and a movement that will always be timeless and moving in their emphasis on health, wholeness, and helping. Through Katherine Ziff, Athens, Ohio, and moral therapy come to life and become inescapably intertwined with our lives!

Samuel T. Gladding, PhD
Chair and Professor, Department of Counseling
Wake Forest University

PREFACE

In 1867 the Ohio legislature laid the foundation for a twenty-year experiment in moral treatment psychiatry at Athens, a small village in the rural southeastern corner of the state. Built to American psychiatry's nineteenth-century gold standard, the Kirkbride plan for moral treatment, the Athens Lunatic Asylum proposed to cure its patients with orderly routines, beautiful views of the countryside, exposure to the arts, a built environment with abundant natural light and plenty of ventilation, outdoor exercise, useful occupation, and personal attention from a physician. Its restorative landscape and efforts to offer humane treatment were a revolution in care for those with mental illness and stand in contrast to hundreds of years of treatment featuring confinement, restraint, and punishment. Nearly a century and a half later, the asylum is making new history as one of the most fully realized examples of the repurposing of old Kirkbride buildings into a university and community resource.

I moved to Athens, Ohio, in 1998. On the first day of my first visit to town, I walked with my son over to The Ridges, the new name for the complex of buildings and landscape that were once the Athens Lunatic Asylum. As we climbed the steep hill to watch bicycle racers rattle over the brick drive around the old asylum buildings, my first impression was of trees. To reach the imposing brick buildings, we walked through a small grove of towering evergreens, remnants of the original landscape planted more than a century ago by landscape gardener George Link and the group of asylum patients who served as his work crew. The buildings and their grounds sit on top of a long and substantial terrace flanking the Hocking River, formed two million years ago in a collision of geology and climate change in southeastern Ohio. If you drive down Route 33 from Columbus, Ohio, toward Athens, just after you pass through Lancaster you will see, as we say in southeastern Ohio, "where the glacier stopped." There the flat terrain gives way to gentle hills that become steeper as you get to Athens, following Highway 33, which crosses the Hocking River twice. As rivers go, the Hocking is relatively young, created as glaciers dammed and then drained the ancient and massive Teays River of central North America. The river's terraces, ninety feet above the present-day riverbed, were formed by the geologic rubble of glacial outwash pushed into the Hocking and deposited downstream alongside the river. Two thousand years ago on the terrace on which The Ridges is located, the Adena built burial mounds deeply imbued with religious, emotional, and psychological meaning.[1] Nearly two millennia later on this site were established the hopes for a healthy, harmonious therapeutic community dedicated to healing persons with mental illness. Ohio University is now the steward of over seven hundred acres of this landscape. Part of the complex originally named the Athens Lunatic Asylum, the land supported the asylum's dairy, orchards, park, lakes, greenhouses, kitchen gardens, piggery, and herds of cattle.

The asylum at Athens was deeply connected with nineteenth-century America's far-reaching demographic changes. With post-war industrialization, the movement of a large proportion of the population to cities, and the decline of an agrarian economy, asylums were expected to serve a humanitarian function and provide a measure of community stability. The pain and suffering endured by Americans in the Civil War inevitably were exhibited in the lives of its survivors: soldiers and their families who were hospitalized in asylums for trauma and grief. In addition, the grim economic times of the Long Depression of 1873–79 triggered mental health crises. All of these dynamics were features of the asylum at Athens. A scholarly discussion about America's two-hundred-year history of asylums has centered on this question: were asylums built to serve communities and preserve social norms or to provide humanitarian care to individuals with mental illness? The truth is that American asylums, including the one at Athens, served both the humanitarian needs of individuals and the social needs of community structures.[2] The Athens asylum, in its moral treatment years, admitted thousands of patients for a wide array of reasons, from a coal miner who was committed for seeking to organize his fellow workers into a labor union to persons who had made attempts to kill themselves and their families to women in need of respite care after childbirth.

A central strand of the moral treatment practiced for twenty years at Athens, as well as in asylums across the United States, is therapeutic place, or the healing properties of a landscape, whether a natural geography or one intentionally shaped.[3] The landscape designer for the Athens asylum, gardener Herman Haerlin of Cincinnati, worked in the nineteenth-century tradition of landscaping pioneered in America by Frederick Law Olmsted: creating a natural wildness that would calm the mind and soothe the soul.[4] The idea of therapeutic, or restorative, landscape has been around for millennia, from at least the time of Asclepius and the Asclepian healing temples built in ancient Greece high above the sea on cliffs and bluffs affording beautiful views.[5] Known also as restorative gardens, therapeutic landscapes have reemerged from time to time, notably in medieval monastic gardens such as that of Bernard of Clairvaux at the hospice of his French monastery.[6] Today in the twenty-first century, the strand has emerged again, flourishing this time along with treatment modalities grounded in nineteenth-century moral treatment and reconceived with new names and disciplines such as wilderness therapy, milieu therapy, creative arts therapies, humanistic psychology, and restorative gardening.[7]

If you take a walk on the dirt roads and paths through the old fields around the Athens Lunatic Asylum buildings today, you will see great drifts of milkweed, *Asclepius syriaca,* a symbolic reminder of the roots of the moral treatment experiment at the Athens Lunatic Asylum. In early summer these tall plants nod with round magenta flower heads, which in August swell into pale green pods that by winter have dried and burst, releasing thousands of seeds that float on silky white threads. They evoke Asclepius, the healer of ancient Greece, who was taking up his work about the time that the Adena were using the grounds of the site of the Athens asylum for sacred purposes.

The research for this book was approved by the Ohio Department of Mental Health, which provided me with access to a wealth of nineteenth-century medical records, including patient commitment documents, the original 1874 medical logs, and files of the writings of patients and their families. I have had the privilege of reading thousands of patient case files and present here those illustrating the conditions and themes underlying the commitment of individuals to the asylum at Athens between 1874 and 1893. Although ultimately doomed by overcrowding and overshadowed by the rise of new models of care, for twenty years the therapeutic community at Athens pursued moral treatment therapy with energy and optimism.

The asylum has been known by eleven different names since it opened in 1874:

TABLE P.I

Names for the institution since its founding

Athens Lunatic Asylum	1868–76
Athens Hospital for the Insane	1876–78
Athens Asylum for the Insane	1878–94
Athens State Hospital	1894–1968
Southeastern Ohio Mental Health Center	1968–69
Athens Mental Health Center	1969–75
Athens Mental Health and Mental Retardation Center	1975–79
Athens Mental Health and Developmental Center	1979–81
Athens Mental Health Center	1981–93
Southeast Psychiatric Hospital	1993–2001
Appalachian Behavioral Healthcare	2001–

Athens Lunatic Asylum, the name under which it opened, is the one used throughout this work. In 1993, the asylum closed and moved to a new and much smaller building directly across the river on its northern banks.[8] The chapters of this book illustrate the moral treatment era (1874–93) at the Athens Lunatic Asylum through stories of tragedy, politics, confusion, struggle, and hope. Drawing upon case histories, medical notes, commitment documents, letters, and reports, each chapter illustrates a facet of the moral treatment experiment at the Athens Lunatic Asylum, including its patients, architecture, politics, therapeutic landscape, and caregivers.

Acknowledgments

This is the first book published on the history of the Athens Lunatic Asylum. Until now, people seeking to learn about the asylum had to search in a variety of works scattered in many places. The general difficulty of gaining a coherent picture of especially the early history has contributed to all kinds of conjecture and supposition, which have served to continue the stigma still associated with mental illness that lingers about the asylum. I hope that this work, by presenting facts and stories of actual events and people, will help dispel rumors and speculation. I have spent eleven years—much longer than I originally thought—researching the asylum, and my work was made possible by the support of many people and organizations.

Particular thanks go to staff of the Ohio University Libraries and its Robert E. and Jean R. Mahn Center for Archives and Special Collections: Doug McCabe, Bill Kimok, Janet Carleton, Judy Connick, and George Bain worked for over a decade with patience, expertise, and enthusiasm to support my work. Janet along with Kelly Broughton made it possible for me to tell the story of the asylum with historical photographs. Others who provided help with the many images are the Athens County Historical Society and Museum, the State Library of Ohio, the Chicago Public Library, the Cosmos Club, the National Archives, and the *Athens Messenger*. The Ohio Historical Society in Columbus, custodian of the original 1874 asylum casebooks, helped provide a unique window into life in the moral treatment years of the asylum. George Eberts, a former employee of the asylum, was an early supporter of my research; Dave Malawista, Sue Foster, and Pam Callahan were also kind enough to share their experience with me.

Much of the material presented here is drawn from patient records, access to which remains restricted because of the patient names associated with the records kept by the asylum. The Ohio Department of Mental Health approved my research (twice— once as doctoral research and again for the book) as one of their projects and provided access to the restricted patient records held by the Mahn Center and the Ohio Historical Society.

Ohio University's Patton College of Education supported my dissertation, out of which grew this book, with a research grant. The Patton College of Education also awarded me a scholarship from the HVFH/Pi Beta Phi Endowment Fund for Graduate Student Support, which gave me time to complete my initial research. I am grateful also to Janice Phelps Williams for her advice and encouragement.

Thanks go to Ohio University Press and to Gillian Berchowitz for making this book a reality. Thanks also to the Athens-Hocking-Vinton 317 Board and the Athens County Convention and Visitors Bureau for their generous support for the production of the book. I also acknowledge the patients, caregivers, families, farmers, builders, craftsmen, communities, elected officials, and administrators who figured in the history of the asylum. I hope I have done them justice.

ONE

THE MORAL TREATMENT EXPERIMENT

"A Magnificent Site Overlooking the Hocking Valley"

On a spring day in 1865, Dr. William Parker Johnson returned home to Athens, Ohio, from the Civil War. He had been mustered out from Camp Dennison in Columbus, Ohio. Three weeks earlier, General Robert E. Lee had surrendered the Confederate Army of Northern Virginia to Lieutenant General Ulysses S. Grant. Dr. Johnson, known to friends and family as Park, was a country doctor. He had enlisted in the Eighteenth Ohio Volunteer Infantry as a physician and finished his war career as head of two post hospitals in Tennessee, where he found a calling as an organizer and administrator. He returned to Athens transformed from country doctor to experienced hospital administrator by his work caring for the ill and wounded of the Kentucky and Tennessee battlefields.

Politics

Men who survived the Civil War returned home to resume their lives; some were shattered in body or mind and others had gained new leadership skills and recognition for heroic achievements. The political careers of Ohio-born presidents Ulysses S. Grant, Rutherford B. Hayes, James Garfield, Benjamin Harrison, and William McKinley were launched by their service as Civil War officers.[1] Dr. Johnson used his war experience and newly developed administrative skills to advance the care of those with mental illness in Ohio by orchestrating the founding of Ohio's fifth state mental hospital, the Athens Lunatic Asylum.

Post–Civil War Ohio was of national significance in the nineteenth-century public mental health care movement sweeping the nation. The Ohio Lunatic Asylum, opened in the state's capital of Columbus in 1838, was the first public asylum west of the Allegheny Mountains.[2] Between 1838 and 1898, Ohio opened seven public asylums to provide mental health care for the state's large and rapidly urbanizing population. All seven were devoted to care based on the newest humanitarian models of mental health care. Some of Ohio's asylum physicians during this period attained national stature, publishing and providing leadership in the newly forming field of American psychiatry. And Ohio in the last quarter of the nineteenth century was an American political and economic powerhouse. Ohio sent five presidents to the White House between 1877 and 1901. Entrepreneurs such as Dr. B. F. Goodrich, Edward Libbey, and John D. Rockefeller established small businesses in Ohio that grew into giant industries. Ohio's natural resources fueled the nation's steel, natural gas, oil, and clay pipe industries, while the state's railways and water transport on Lake Erie and the Ohio River provided a dense network of transportation between the East and the rapidly expanding markets of the West.[3]

In contrast to the urban centers of Cincinnati, Columbus, Toledo, Dayton, and Cleveland, Athens remains even today a small village in a remote rural corner of Ohio. Established in 1804 by the General Assembly of Ohio as the home for Ohio University, Athens was surveyed in 1795 by the Ohio Company, whose associates were among those who settled the midwestern wilderness under the Ordinance of the Northwest Territory, 1787.[4] The village's 1870 population of seventeen hundred persons and its isolated location in the steep, forested foothills at the edge of the Appalachian Mountains made it an extraordinary choice for the location of Ohio's fifth state asylum.

Dr. Johnson's first year as a war doctor was difficult. He was often depressed and in despair about alleviating the human misery created by war, as he wrote to his wife, Julia, in Athens from Camp Jefferson at Bacon Creek, Kentucky, in June 1861:

> My shoulders are pretty broad and I guess I can go on
> awhile although I hope our regiment will not continue long
> in its distressed condition. I thought yesterday we were
> about through with measles but found seven new cases
> today. The chances for making the sick men comfortable

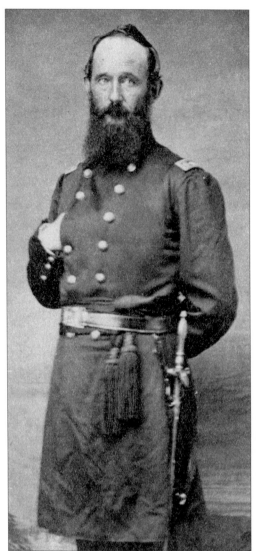

FIGURE 1.1 Dr. William Parker ("Parks") Johnson, brigade surgeon in the Eighteenth Ohio Infantry. He was elected to the Ohio legislature in 1864 while serving in the Union Army. *Courtesy of the Mahn Center for Archives and Special Collections, Ohio University Libraries.*

FIGURE 1.2 Julia Blackstone Johnson, wife of Dr. William Parker Johnson. *Courtesy of the Mahn Center for Archives and Special Collections, Ohio University Libraries.*

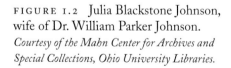
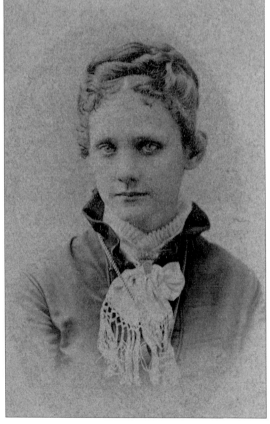

are miserable and I dread the consequences very much—we have lost but one case yet. We have on hand now a number very sick and several will have to die I fear. People have little idea of the horrors of war—it is not easy to be on a battlefield however I do not think it best to distress your tender feelings with any particulars and I presume it is not best for you to mention anything about the facts I have stated as so many of the Athens people have friends here. . . . [W]hen will this accursed war be at an end?[5]

But Dr. Johnson persisted and later wrote Julia of his success in organizing his work. His letters suggest that his interest in mental health care may have been a result of his observations of soldiers in distress for no apparent physical reason and his puzzlement as to how to treat them in his hospitals.

It is a matter of astonishment how much one man can do when he goes at it with a will. I would not have believed a month since that it were possible for one (me) to do what I have done for the past two or three months. . . . It will have at least one good effect in learning me to be ready to do the right thing at the right time. I have my labors so systematized that I have a time for each only and aim to discharge it just at the proper time. I have got the men learned so that there is a time set apart for each particular entry. For instance all who are on the complaining order in camp must make their complaints known between the hours of light and ten in the morning. . . . One of my great perplexities is what to do with men who claim to be sick and yet present no outward symptoms of disease.[6]

Despite a massive workload, diarrhea, and occasional bouts of depression, Dr. Johnson came to appreciate his work. From Tullahoma, Tennessee, he wrote that while he worried constantly about his family and missed the comforts of home, he preferred the regularity of life as an army physician to working in the hills of Appalachian Ohio as a country doctor:

Doctor Mills got sad news from home last night. One of his children died and his wife and his three other children were all very sick with scarlet fever. Poor fellow he is almost distracted. He applied today for leave of absence but could not obtain it. I have urged him to go anyhow. . . .

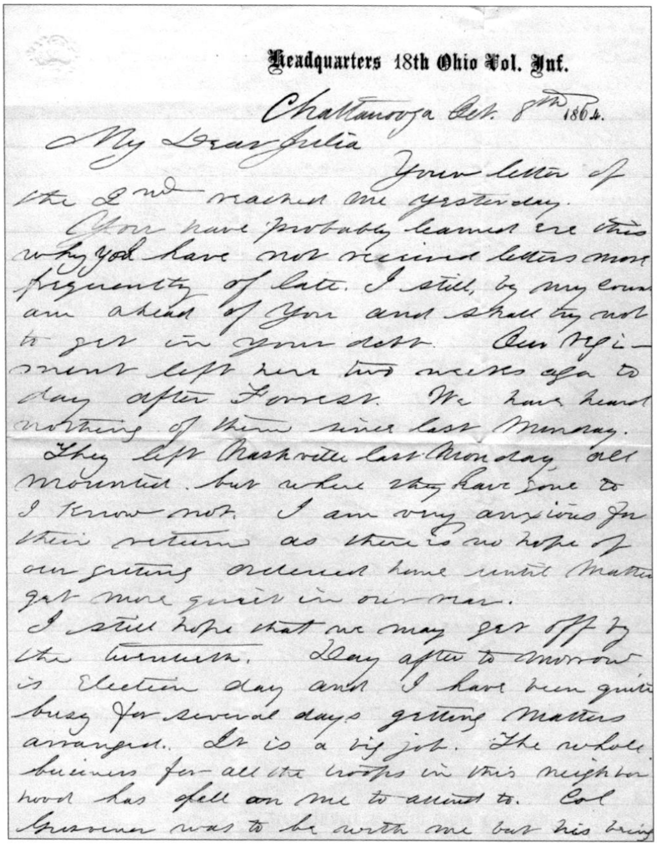

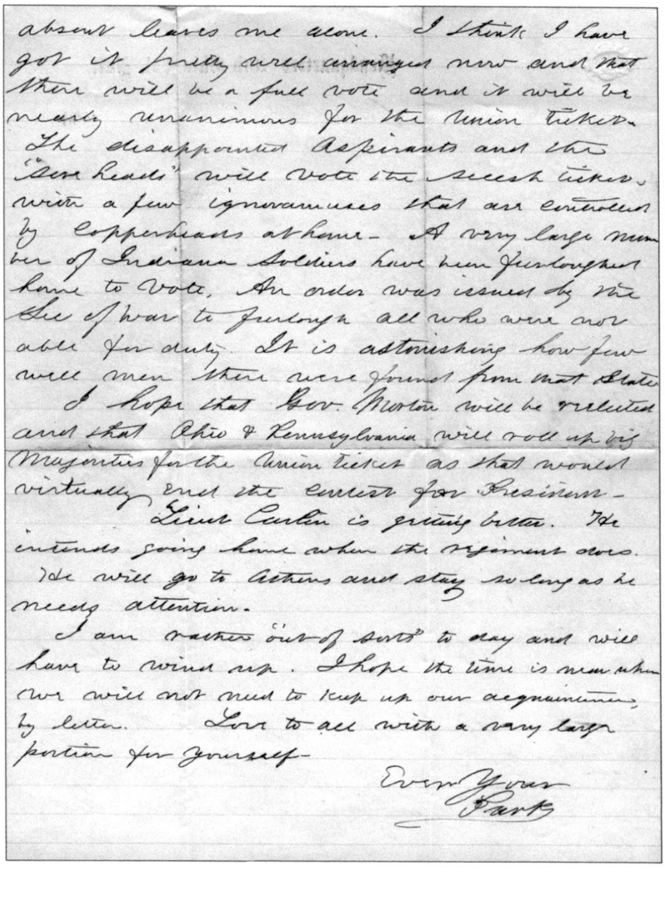

FIGURE 1.3 Letter to his wife, Julia, from Dr. William Parker Johnson, Athens physician and head of two Union post hospitals in Tennessee. An Ohio legislator, Dr. Johnson orchestrated the founding of the new asylum in 1867 and its location in Athens. While away at war, he wrote often to Julia. In this letter, he discusses the 1864 presidential election. *Courtesy of the Mahn Center for Archives and Special Collections, Ohio University Libraries.*

It is the one real drawback to being a soldier the constant anxiety about the loved ones at home. So far as the mere labor is concerned, I would rather occupy my present position than return to my old practice over the Athens County hills. I can be more regular in my meals (if they are sometimes very poor) and lose less sleep than in my old practice at home but nothing can compensate for the loss of the endearments at home and its precious treasures.[7]

Late in 1863, Johnson was given greater administrative responsibility. Writing to Julia from Murfreesboro, Tennessee, he described his new work and reflected again on the horrors of war:

I mentioned in my letter to your father that I had been put in charge of a Post Hospital here. I have got it fitted up very comfortably and all men (except some who were slightly wounded sent to Nashville) in it. Today I received orders to take another Hospital under my charge. I protested against both for the reason that I already had enough to do and also for the reason that it was in such a miserable condition. I was informed that that was the reason that it was put in my charge so that its condition might be improved. . . . War has its Glories but it has also its thousand horrors and human tortures that would sicken any feeling heart. I have often wished to see a big battle but I pray to God that I may never witness again such scenes as I have had to for the last two weeks. I have no desire to horrify you with any attempt at a description and could not give the subject justice should I attempt it.[8]

Just before he returned to Athens from the war, Dr. Johnson was elected to the Ohio legislature, where in 1867 he orchestrated the founding of the Athens Lunatic Asylum. Having learned well his organizational lessons from his war work, Johnson did "the right things at the right time" to secure state approval for a new asylum and ensure its location at Athens. First he helped a legislator from a nearby county craft a resolution in the General Assembly directing Ohio's Committee on Benevolent Institutions to look into the needs of those with mental illness in Ohio. The resolution passed in 1866. Second, as chair of the Committee on Benevolent Institutions, Johnson solicited from the state medical society, of which he was a member, reports to the legislature supporting the need for more institutions to serve those judged insane. Finally, Johnson prepared a bill authorizing the construction of the fifth state asylum. This bill, entitled "An act to provide for the erection of an additional lunatic asylum," passed in 1866 and became a law in 1867. Finally, in a deft political move, Johnson saw to it that Athens businessman E. H. Moore was appointed by the governor as one of three trustees of the new asylum charged with choosing its location. Moore organized the Athens community to collect money for the purchase of the site and offer it free to the state. After considering more than thirty locations, it came as no surprise to anyone that the trustees settled upon Athens.

The village of Athens celebrated the laying of the cornerstone of its asylum with a parade of nearly ten thousand persons. The new institution coming to town was of great economic and political importance to its residents, who staged an enormous celebration. On Thursday, November 5, 1868, at two o'clock in the afternoon, one thousand Masons from all over Ohio, a brass band, two church choirs, judges, the mayor of Athens, the village council, hundreds of townspeople, and thousands of supporters from other areas marched down a long hill across the old South Bridge spanning the Hockhocking River[9] and up the great hill to the asylum grounds.[10] Ohio's fifth state-supported asylum to treat persons with mental illness was to be a Kirkbride hospital, the gold standard for Victorian-era mental hospitals. Kirkbride hospitals were built to the most rigorous specifications of moral treatment, the prevailing psychiatric treatment of the time.

The Kirkbride Plan

Dr. Thomas Kirkbride's interpretation of moral treatment, developed at the Pennsylvania Hospital for the Insane, was the crown jewel of nineteenth-century American psychiatry.[11] He proposed that mental illness was curable, that physical punishment and restraints should be abolished, that treatment of those with mental illness as though they were capable of rational behavior was curative, and that a system of routines and diversions in a restful and supportive setting was therapeutic. Dr. Philippe Pinel, physician for two asylums in Paris, touched off the moral treatment movement in 1795 when he allegedly removed chains from his patients and undertook humane, compassionate, and supportive care. He dubbed his method *traitement morale,* meaning ethical, honorable treatment. This approach was a radical alternative to well-established aggressive, punitive tactics of curing mental illness with punishment and restraints. A year later, in 1796, William Tuke, a Quaker tea merchant, opened the York Retreat for persons with mental illness, using kindness, reason, and a family atmosphere rather than the medical treatments of the time.[12]

Nineteenth-century asylum physicians dedicated to moral treatment believed that mental illness was curable through proper habits and a regular, healthy life. Dr. William H. Holden, superintendent of the Athens Lunatic Asylum, described moral treatment in his 1879 annual report to the Board of Trustees:

> Under the head of moral treatment must be considered all those means that tend to lead the mind into a normal and healthy channel, and direct the thoughts, as much as possible, in another course, remote from their delusions. See your patients frequently; talk to them, give them kind words and pleasant looks; encourage them as much as possible. Give them moderate exercise. Walking, riding, and driving in the open air have a tendency to break the monotony of asylum life and add to the comfort and happiness of the patient. Voluntary exercise is indicative of improvement and should be encouraged. Occupation engrosses the mind and withdraws it from empty longings and illusions of the imagination.[13]

Psychiatry placed great faith in the curative possibilities offered by the physical setting and social influences of the asylum; indeed, a Kirkbride hospital is a visual and architectural record of nineteenth-century psychiatry's tenets. Kirkbride's guidelines for the construction and operation of hospitals for the insane were adopted in 1851 by the Association of Medical Superintendents of American Institutions for the Insane.[14] The guidelines, almost unimaginable by today's standards of inpatient care for persons with mental illness, were devoted to the landscape and the design and construction of the building. Nearly eighty asylums were built in America to the specifications of the Kirkbride plan, most of them between 1848 and 1890. From Taunton State Hospital (completed in 1854) in Massachusetts, Jackson State Hospital (1855) in Mississippi, Mendota State Hospital (1860) in Wisconsin, Dixmont State Hospital (1852) in Pennsylvania, Worcester State Hospital (1877) in Massachusetts, Napa State Hospital (1875) in California, and Terrell State Hospital (1885) in Texas to Traverse City State

Hospital (1885) in Michigan, states embarked on construction of Kirkbride asylums on a massive scale.[15]

Dr. Kirkbride suggested that hospitals should be located in the country and have at least fifty acres devoted to gardens and pleasure grounds for patients with at least another fifty acres for farming and other uses. "The building should be in a healthful, pleasant, and fertile district of the country; the land chosen should be of good quality and easily tilled; the surrounding scenery should be varied and attractive, and the neighborhood should possess numerous objects of an agreeable and interesting character."[16] To bring light and cheer to each wing of the hospital, each floor should have an atrium with plants, birds and fountains:

> Leaving on each side (of each wing) an open space of
> ten or twelve feet, with movable glazed sash extending
> from near the floor to the ceiling, and which may
> either be accessible to the patients, or be protected by
> ornamental open wire work on a line with the corridor;
> this arrangement gives nearly every advantage of light,
> air, and scenery. Behind such a screen, even in the most
> excited wards, may be placed with entire security, the most
> beautiful evergreen and flowering plants, singing birds, jets
> of water, and various other objects, the contemplation of
> which can not fail to have a pleasant and soothing effect
> upon every class of patients.[17]

The Kirkbride plan called for twelve-foot ceilings in all the patient wards with sixteen-foot ceilings in the central administrative section. Hospital residential corridors should be at least twelve feet wide, with those of the central building sixteen feet wide. Spacious corridors and high ceilings facilitated good ventilation; indeed, the Athens asylum was situated so as to take advantage of the prevailing breeze through the large and plentiful windows.[18] The parlors and other large rooms on each floor of a Kirkbride hospital were each twenty feet square. Patient bedrooms were kept small enough (about a hundred square feet) so that their dimensions would not encourage placement of two patients in the same room:

> The single chambers for patients should be made as large
> as can be well brought about, provided their dimensions are
> not so great as to lead to two patients being placed in the
> same room, which ought not to be allowed. Nine feet front

by eleven feet deep will probably be adopted as the best size, although eight by ten is admissible, and has the advantage that when not larger than this, two patients are not likely to be put into one room. If the rooms are larger, this is almost certain to be done whenever a hospital becomes crowded, and it is really never either proper or safe, to have two insane patients sleep in the same room without an attendant in it, or in an adjoining one. Great convenience will be found in having in each ward at least one chamber of the size of two single rooms, for the use of a patient with a special attendant, or in cases of severe illness.[19]

Compassionate, supportive treatment of those with mental illness was a sea change, a manifestation of the great Victorian impulse to provide systematic, decent public care for vulnerable individuals—those with mental illness, orphans, the poor, and persons in need of medical care.[20] The nineteenth century in America ushered in a national outpouring of support for social institutions: medical hospitals, mental hospitals, universities, public schools, penitentiaries, YMCA and YWCAs, the Red Cross, orphanages, settlement houses, schools for blind persons, and schools for deaf persons. This groundswell of support rose in response to the needs of family, community, and industry. With postwar industrialization, the decline of an agrarian economy, and the rise of cities, asylums and other institutions were expected to serve a humanitarian function and also to provide a measure of social stability. By today's standards, this charity movement led by social reformers, many of them women, was paternalistic, selective, and moralistic. Many of the major community institutions in America today were invented in the nineteenth century to bring order to or meet social needs created by industrialization and urbanization of American life.[21] Orphanages, libraries, public schools, colleges and universities, health clinics, penitentiaries, parks, hospitals, and asylums for those with mental illness were among the institutions developed by states working with networks of community organizations and social reformers to alleviate poor living conditions in nineteenth-century American towns and cities.

Discussion among asylum scholars, former asylum patients, historians, and sociologists about the role and function of asylums has historically been dominated by debates about whether asylums were built to serve a humanitarian purpose or to act as an instrument of social control. Andrew Scull has recentered the hundred-year debate by describing asylums as a means for reinforcing social

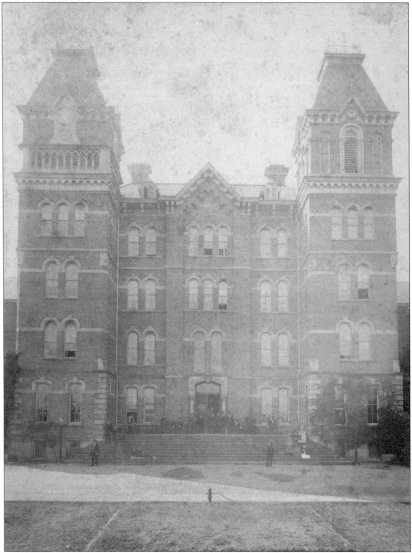

conformity while acknowledging the very real needs experienced by families attempting to cope with mental illness.[22]

The movement for humanitarian care and public services blossomed in Ohio in the mid-nineteenth century, a response to the humanitarian impulse and the needs of a rapidly industrializing state. Across Ohio, public schools were established, libraries were begun, institutions were founded to serve orphans and persons with physical disabilities, and state hospitals were established for those with mental illness. Ohio built five Kirkbride hospitals in the nineteenth century, more than any other state except Massachusetts, which also had five. Ohio was the second state (after Massachusetts) to establish a Board of State Charities to provide oversight over Ohio's state benevolent and correctional institutions. Charged with investigating and reporting on the condition of state benevolent and correctional institutions, the board, whose members served without compensation, was an advocate for persons with mental illness. The board routinely investigated complaints about asylums and documented conditions for the mentally ill who resided in jails or county infirmaries or, in some tragic cases, were kept naked in barnyards or locked in family basements. Governor Rutherford B. Hayes praised the board's efforts, noting that "they have faithfully performed the thankless task of investigating and reporting the defects in the system . . . of our charitable and penal laws."[23]

The Athens Lunatic Asylum was the last built of Ohio's Kirkbride hospitals. Its architecture reflected its dedication to the national moral treatment experiment. Featuring a central section with a two long stepped-back wings, the asylum had three levels with a

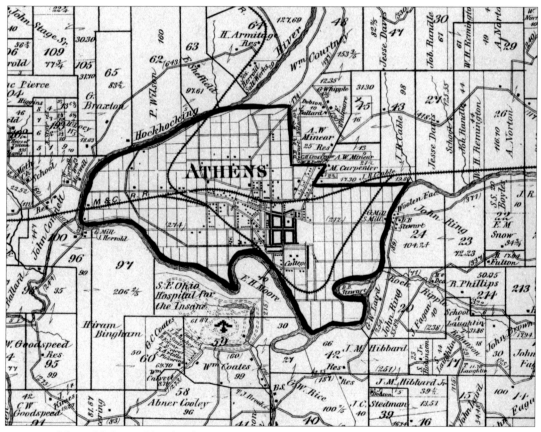

FIGURE 1.5 Map of Athens, Ohio (1875), showing the location of the asylum southwest of the Hockhocking River. The asylum is labeled "S.E. Ohio Hospital for the Insane." The South Bridge, northeast of the hospital, connected the village and the asylum. Originally published in D. J. Lake, *Atlas of Athens County, Ohio. Courtesy of the Mahn Center for Archives and Special Collections, Ohio University Libraries.*

central administrative core of four levels, an attic, and a cellar. Male patients were housed in the east wing, women in the west wing. The central section housed offices and living quarters for professional staff, storerooms, visiting rooms for patients to receive visitors, a parlor, and a ballroom. The original structure (completed in 1874) contained 544 rooms. Patients were housed in 450 rooms; the asylum was designed to accommodate 252 patients in single bedrooms and an additional 290 in dormitory-style rooms. Food was transported from the kitchens along a small basement railroad and lifted upstairs by dumbwaiters to individual wards. The facility was heated by six coal-fired steam boilers in a separate rear building.[24]

The site, which eventually encompassed over a thousand acres, began in 1867 with 150 acres on a bluff across the Hockhocking River from Athens. Eighteen and a half million bricks used for construction of the huge building were made by hand on the site

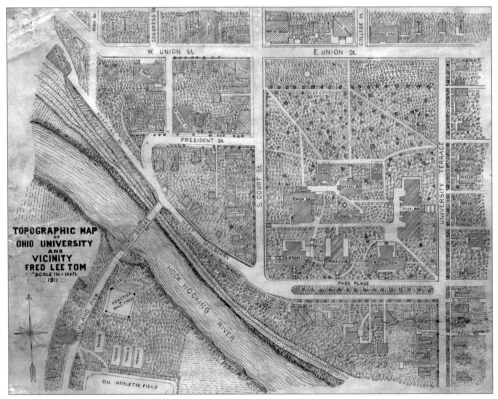

FIGURE 1.6 Map of Ohio University (1911) showing the South Bridge, northeast of the hospital, connecting the village of Athens and the asylum. In 1889, the asylum and the village collaborated to build Hospital Street *(upper left)* to provide paved access to the train depot. The road was built entirely by asylum employees and patients on right-of-way acquired by the village. Fred Lee Tom, topographic map of Ohio University and vicinity (hand-drawn map, 1911), used with permission courtesy of Fred C. Tom. *Courtesy of the Mahn Center for Archives and Special Collections, Ohio University Libraries.*

using clay from the asylum's grounds. Its hundreds of windows featured protective bars disguised as ornate wrought iron circles. The asylum was "situated upon a high plateau of land about a mile distant from the town of Athens, the river Hockhocking winding in its circuitous course through the valley between the asylum and town. The farm belonging to it comprises about one hundred and fifty acres, broken in its surface, somewhat wooded."[25]

Humanitarian Need and Social Control

On New Year's Day in 1874, the asylum opened its doors to patients, six months later than had been planned. Built to care for 542 patients, within six years it housed 633 patients from twenty-nine counties in southeastern Ohio, as well as "overflow" patients from Columbus State Hospital, which was destroyed by fire in 1868. Rebuilt along the Kirkbride plan, the Columbus asylum reopened in 1877, relieving some of the crowding at Athens. From its beginning, though, the asylum at Athens was built to accommodate twice the number of patients recommended by Kirkbride: "Two hundred and fifty will be found about as many as the medical superintendent can visit properly every day, or nearly every day, in addition to the performance of his other duties."[26]

Patients came from all walks of life. Most of the men were farmers from southeastern Ohio. There were also miners, machinists, railroad hands, school superintendents, schoolteachers, physicians, lawyers, engineers, students, clerks, merchants, saloonkeepers, hotelkeepers, glassblowers, carpenters, shoemakers, brewers, bakers, tailors, bookbinders, and printers. The occupations of female patients were not documented in the asylum's annual reports—only women's status as to whether they were married, widowed, or single. Each admission to the asylum was assigned a number; persons admitted more than once were given a new number each time they were admitted. The asylum used this numbering system until at least the 1950s.

Commitment documents and the asylum's only surviving casebooks, large leather-bound volumes recording the admission and progress of patients admitted in 1874, reveal detailed stories. For some, the Athens Lunatic Asylum served a humanitarian function, providing respite for families desperate for help in caring for their mentally ill relatives and a safe haven for many patients. For others, the asylum was an agent of control, acting to preserve dominant economic interests and the moral sensibilities of a late Victorian-era community.

The asylum case records contain many examples of men and women in critical need of care. For example, Female Patient 454 was first hospitalized at age forty-eight, pregnant with her seventh child. "Whipped" by her husband and having just lost her sisters to consumption, she had her first "attack" of insanity. Four years later, at age fifty-two with seven children to care for, an abusive spouse to contend with, and in ill health, the asylum again provided respite care for her as Female Patient 1175.[27]

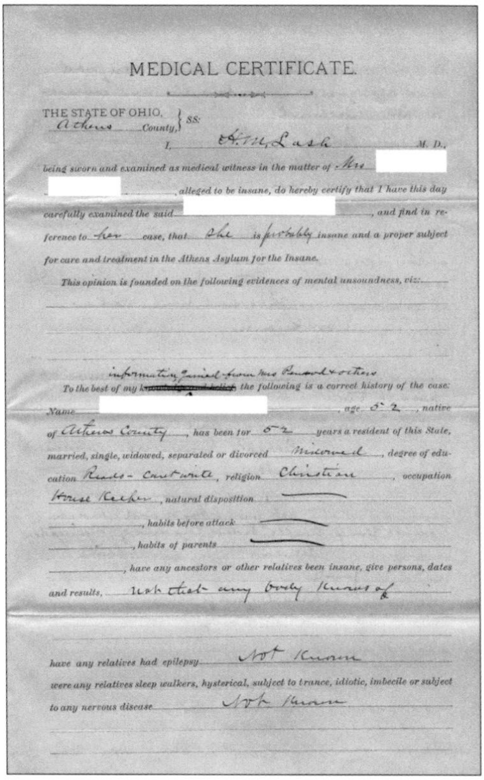

MEDICAL CERTIFICATE.

THE STATE OF OHIO, Athens County, } SS:

I, H. M. Lash M. D., being sworn and examined as medical witness in the matter of Mrs [redacted] [redacted], alleged to be insane, do hereby certify that I have this day carefully examined the said [redacted], and find in reference to her case, that she is probably insane and a proper subject for care and treatment in the Athens Asylum for the Insane.

This opinion is founded on the following evidences of mental unsoundness, viz:

To the best of my ~~knowledge and belief~~ information gained from Mrs [illegible] & others the following is a correct history of the case:

Name [redacted], age 52, native of Athens County, has been for 52 years a resident of this State, married, single, widowed, separated or divorced Married, degree of education Reads - Cant write, religion Christian, occupation House Keeper, natural disposition —, habits before attack —, habits of parents —, have any ancestors or other relatives been insane, give persons, dates and results, Not that any body knows of

have any relatives had epilepsy Not Known

were any relatives sleep walkers, hysterical, subject to trance, idiotic, imbecile or subject to any nervous disease Not Known

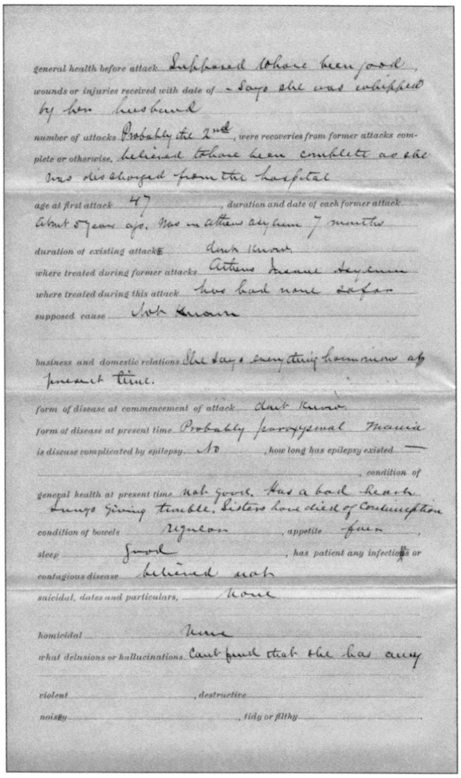

general health before attack Supposed to have been good, wounds or injuries received with date of - Says she was whipped by her husband

number of attacks Probably the 2nd, were recoveries from former attacks complete or otherwise, believed to have been complete as she was discharged from the hospital

age at first attack 47, duration and date of each former attack About 5 years ago. Was in Athens asylum 7 months

duration of existing attacks dont know

where treated during former attacks Athens Insane Asylum

where treated during this attack has had none so far

supposed cause Not Known

business and domestic relations She says everything harmonious at present time.

form of disease at commencement of attack dont know

form of disease at present time Probably paroxysmal Mania

is disease complicated by epilepsy No, how long has epilepsy existed —, condition of general health at present time not good. Has a bad heart Lungs giving trouble. Sisters have died of Consumption

condition of bowels regular, appetite fair, sleep good, has patient any infectious or contagious disease believed not

suicidal, dates and particulars, None

homicidal None

what delusions or hallucinations Cant find that she has any

violent, destructive

noisy, tidy or filthy.

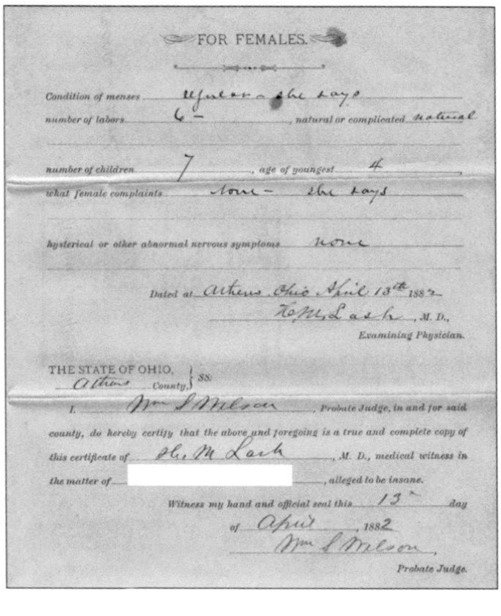

FOR FEMALES.

Condition of menses regular - she says

number of labors 6 -, natural or complicated natural

number of children 7, age of youngest 4,

what female complaints None - she says

hysterical or other abnormal nervous symptoms none

Dated at Athens Ohio April 13th 1882

H. M. Lash, M. D., Examining Physician.

THE STATE OF OHIO, Athens County, } SS:

I, Wm S Nelson, Probate Judge, in and for said county, do hereby certify that the above and foregoing is a true and complete copy of this certificate of H. M. Lash, M. D., medical witness in the matter of [redacted], alleged to be insane.

Witness my hand and official seal this 13th day of April, 1882

Wm S Nelson, Probate Judge.

FIGURE 1.7 Medical certificate presented to probate court for the purpose of committing Female Patient 1175. *Courtesy of the Mahn Center for Archives and Special Collections, Ohio University Libraries.*

Female Patient 1296, burdened with worries and delusions, was admitted in the summer of 1883 when she was thirty-four years old. She and her young daughter lived with her mother in a farming community. The committing physician wrote of her:

> She has Insomnia and is unreasonable in conversation. [She has] ill feeling toward her mother and daughter whom she has always loved and cared for. She has constant fear of coming to poverty and dying in the poorhouse. She has had a great deal of trouble with business and domestic relations. Has paroxysms of scolding and using profane language. Very nervous, wakeful and anxious about business. General health is not good. . . . She has threatened to put her child out of the way and imagines her physician wants to marry her, if she was only rid of her little girl.[28]

Male Patient 35, a saddler from Columbus, Ohio, was despondent over having lost money through a business transaction and tried to hang himself several times. His wife, worried about his well-being and safety, took him before the county probate judge for commitment, and he was admitted to the Athens asylum. Fifteen months later, deemed recovered, he was taken home by his wife.[29]

Asylums have always served community needs for social stability, and the Athens asylum was no different. Patients' rights were nonexistent in the nineteenth century. An Ohio citizen could be involuntarily committed upon the recommendation of the county probate judge and the written word of a physician that the patient was insane. The judge forwarded his recommendation for commitment along with the medical certificate to the superintendent of the state asylum, who made the decision whether or not to hospitalize. Occasionally a probate judge attached with his legal forms a handwritten note asking for special consideration on behalf of family or community.

A judge from the Ohio River town of Belpre took the unusual step of including with commitment papers a two-page letter asking for help from the asylum superintendent dealing with a patient recently released from the asylum. Upon his release, this former patient did something to generate a warrant for his arrest, but the sheriff failed to arrest him before the warrant expired, and for this reason he could not be confined in jail, much to the annoyance of the community. "The Sheriff failed to arrest _____ within the life of the writ but then did so after which the Probate Judge was absent. . . . I do not know what the end of it will be. . . . [T]he people of Belpre are very much annoyed and if the reports I hear are true something must be done."[30]

Some patients were hospitalized because they exhibited behavior considered bizarre or improper. An Athens family committed one of its daughters after fetching her home from a brothel in Cincinnati. Male Patient 318, a fifty-one-year-old tailor admitted in 1874, was committed for painting morbid pictures. The medical witness to the probate court noted, "The history of his case is as follows: A tailor by trade, he indulges in painting all kinds of objects representing his morbid imagination which are in contradiction with his intelligent countenance. Duration not known. Has never made attempts of violence upon himself nor upon others. He is peaceable."[31]

Public officials in the coalfields of the Hocking River valley used the asylum at Athens on at least one occasion to try to prevent the spread of labor unions. In 1887, a coal miner became Male Patient 1945 in the Athens asylum because he was trying to organize a labor union.[32] Wrote the committing physician, "His talk is constantly in regard to the Knights of Labor. He imagines it is his especial business to organize said society. Over-study about labor organizations is the cause of his insanity."[33] The man's efforts to form a labor union were quickly extinguished by the local judge and a physician willing to attest to his insanity.

Hospitalization was also a solution for the community problem of what to do with homeless men, or "tramps." Nineteenth-century homeless men were viewed as a threat to the social order because they did not work for a living. Robert Frost's turn-of-the-century poem *The Death of the Hired Man* offers a gentle interpretation of homeless men who wander when the weather is fine and return to employers in the winter in need of shelter, who cannot be depended on to complete jobs and talk in jumbles.[34] But the general opinion of tramps in the late nineteenth century was much harsher; they were considered a challenge to the Victorian social order propped up by ideals of work and family, of which the tramp had a commitment to neither. Governor Thomas Young referred in his annual message to the "formidable and dangerous element of society known as tramps."[35] The *Athens Messenger* reported in 1880 that Cincinnati police shot and killed a tramp when he resisted arrest for verbally insulting several ladies.[36]

The Athens asylum took in tramps. Male Patient 1675 was hospitalized in 1885. His age was unknown, though he was known to be a native of France. His occupation was listed as "tramp," and the medical witness, Athens physician Dr. J. A. Frame, noted that he slept well, his bowels were regular and his appetite good, he was quiet, and he was neither violent nor destructive. Dr. Frame wrote that he "imagines he is very rich. And that he is thousands of years old."[37]

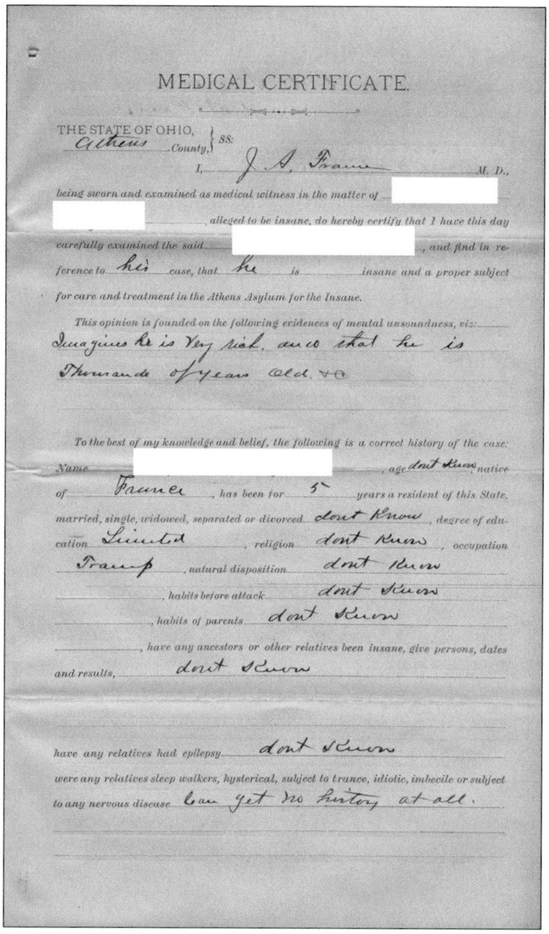

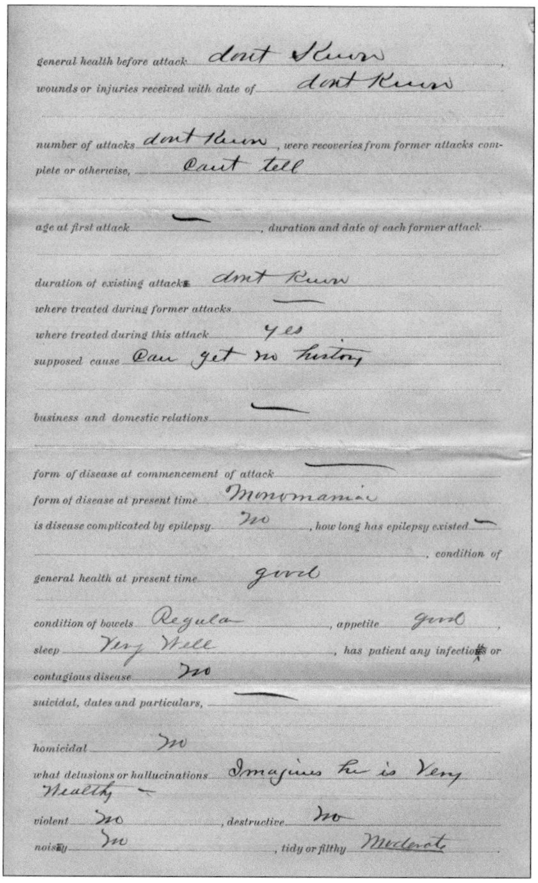

FIGURE 1.8 Medical certificate presented to probate court for the purpose of committing Male Patient 1675. *Courtesy of the Mahn Center for Archives and Special Collections, Ohio University Libraries.*

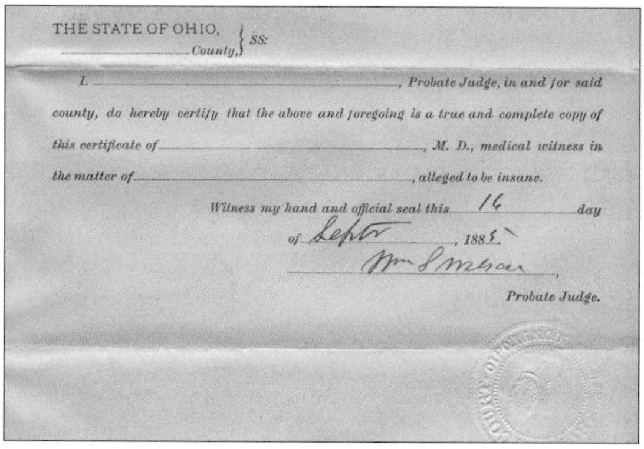

Another tramp, born in Germany, was one of the asylum's earliest patients. Dr. B. Raymond wrote of the wretched condition in which Male Patient 319 was found: "The history of his case is as follows: He was found some years ago walking the road back and forward. People in the neighborhood became affright of him. He was taken up, found in a starving condition. He refuses to speak. He writes in German. The duration is unknown. The patient is free from infectious disease and vermin. He wallers in his excrements."[38]

Although the Civil War produced presidents and community leaders, the massive trauma endured by the nation inevitably exhibited itself in the lives of the war's survivors. The weaponry used in the Civil War introduced a new and higher level of lethality, with the rifled musket and minié ball expanding the killing range of the infantry soldier from fifty to a hundred yards to five hundred yards. Disease claimed twice as many as those who died in combat.[39] The result was a war with massive casualties: 620,000 soldiers and 50,000 civilians. Post-traumatic stress disorder, known from World War I forward as combat fatigue, battle shock, or combat stress reaction, was not diagnosed or defined during the Civil War, but its soldiers could not avoid the effects of war.[40] Civil War physicians referred to stragglers, soldiers afflicted with nostalgia, and soldier's heart. Stragglers were soldiers who sat trembling and clutching their weapons, staring into the distance, exhibiting a startle response at any loud sound, and incapable of engaging in battle. At Antietam, for instance, a third of the Confederates were labeled "stragglers."[41] Nostalgia, a term devised by a seventeenth-century Swiss physician, was characterized by homesickness and defiant aggression, which generally disappeared as soldiers began to prepare for battle, thus triggering the production of adrenaline and other stress hormones in their bodies. Soldier's heart was a cardiac disorder featuring very high heart rates, palpitations, and inability to perform physical work. The asylum at Athens admitted Civil War veterans who suffered from the war's emotional and physical trauma. Some mothers and fathers of men killed in the war were committed because of the trauma of their loss.

Finally, Ohioans suffered during the six-year Long Depression. Triggered by the Panic of 1873, this period of economic decline wreaked havoc across the United States, bankrupting railroads, destroying businesses, and raising unemployment to 14 percent. In Ohio, Governor Edward Noyes devoted his inaugural address in 1873 to the economic disaster, outlining its effects on Ohioans:

A few months ago, that undefinable but tremendous power, called a money panic, imparted a violent shock to the whole industrial and property system of the country.

The well-considered plans and calculations of all men engaged in active business, or in the exertion of active labor, were suddenly and thoroughly deranged. In the universal business anarchy that ensued, the minds of men became more or less bewildered, so that few among them were able distinctly to see their way, or know what to do or what to omit, even through the brief futurity of a single week. All values and all incomes were instantly and deeply depressed. There was not a farmer, a manufacturer, a merchant, a mechanic, or a laborer, who did not feel that he was less able to meet his engagements or pay his taxes than he had been before. The distressful effect of this state of things was felt by all, but it was more grievously felt by the great body of the laboring people, because it touched them at the vital point of subsistence.[42]

As a result of this economic disaster, when the asylum at Athens opened in 1874 many of its first patients were men and women depressed and suicidal about business failure and highly anxious with fears of poverty and want.

The work to create the Athens Lunatic Asylum began three years after the end of the Civil War, and hopes were high for this new institution. Its relatively small size, compared to its contemporary asylums in America and Europe, was considered a favorable point. "Large as it really is," wrote Dr. Richard Gundry (superintendent of the Southern Asylum at Cincinnati) of its room for 570 patients, "it is eclipsed by several in extent and capacity. In New York, the asylum at Utica, with its 800 patients; the New York city asylum, with its 1400 patients; in France La Salpetriere, with its 1400 patients. . . . [I]n England, Colney Hatch or Hanwell, each having more than 1000 inmates."[43] The services of Dr. Gundry had been secured by the Athens asylum trustees for advice and assistance in completing the construction of the Athens facility. He continued in his 1872 report to the newly formed Board of Trustees of the Athens Lunatic Asylum to stress the Kirkbride model's design preference for smaller asylums and the superiority of the asylum at Athens in this regard: "And indeed, while the enormous size of such institutions may be defended on the ground of economy in administration . . . it must be always borne in mind that the true interests of the insane would be better served by smaller institutions and more of them. . . . I repeat that few if any institutions, within my knowledge, will surpass this in the essential and fundamental requirements of all such buildings—the proportion of space, light and air to each patient."[44]

Superintendents of the asylum at Athens were national leaders in limiting patient restraints, a departure from standard nineteenth-century American asylum practice. Ohio asylum superintendents debated their use, and at Athens superintendents consistently provided leadership for a national movement limiting patient restraint.[45] Mechanical restraints such as straps and mittens, chemical restraints to control behavior, manual restraint provided by attendants, locked doors, and seclusion were used infrequently at Athens during the moral treatment years.[46] In his 1872 report to the board, Dr. Gundry advised against constructing strong rooms where "excited" patients would be held when uncontrollable, advocating instead a small ward of individual rooms for such patients, to be "made as cheerful as for any other patients but so constructed as to resist the violence and mischief of the most excited."[47] Dr. Rutter, superintendent in 1877, commented in 1880 on the open-door practice:

> Upon reassuming the duties of Superintendent, I was
> highly gratified to find that the open-doors system in some
> of the wards had been continued during my absence. It
> was, as some of you will doubtless remember, with many
> fears and some misgivings that I took the pioneer step in
> Ohio by removing the locks from some of the wards, and
> permitting full liberty to the patients they contained. That
> it was not ill-considered or reckless has been proved by
> the complete success of the experiment and it is a pleasure
> to add that in my opinion the system can be extended
> until comparatively few of our six hundred patients will be
> behind locks and bars.[48]

While other Ohio asylum physicians argued for the use of restraints as a benevolent practice, Athens superintendents during the moral treatment years believed that restraints were at odds with moral treatment and provided transparency to the public on their limited use through the annual reports of the Board of Trustees.[49]

The architecture of the Athens asylum was central to the moral treatment curative schema. Its light-filled rooms, wide corridors,

Victorian reception parlors, windows situated to provide patients with beautiful and peaceful views of the landscape, ventilation powered by two enormous state-of-the-art brass basement fans manufactured in Pittsburgh, iron protective window grilles disguised as decorative mandalas, wards designed to segregate patients by their levels of disruptive behavior, and elimination of "strong rooms" were all thought vital to the treatment and cure of patients there. Daylight itself was considered curative, as described in near-reverent language by Ohio's Board of State Charities in the 1880 annual report to the governor: "Light is not only cheap, it is a civilizer. Light is healthful, light is good in every way."[50] Flowers, raised in a glass conservatory, were abundant year-round. Superintendent W. H. Holden noted with satisfaction the floral supply: "The florist's department, during the past year, has been exceedingly satisfactory, giving us a full supply of flowers for the general household, besides having abundance for the grounds where sufficiently completed to receive them. We have repaired our conservatory by a complete relaying of the glass. . . . [I]t is now in a better condition than ever before for the recuperation and preservation, through the winter, of the exotics and indigenous plants, in which the patients and visitors so much delight."[51]

Superintendents and trustees during the asylum's moral treatment years were eager to transform the asylum's steep hills and wet bottomlands into beautiful, curative scenery. The grounds were considered to offer great natural beauties needing only grading and filling. This work, requiring blasting and shoveling massive amounts of rock and dirt into pans pulled by teams of horses and mules, was accomplished over twenty years with labor provided by male patients and paid townsmen. Superintendent Clarke requested eight thousand dollars in 1878 from the state for grading and lake improvements; the trustees wrote to the governor that "we have no hesitancy in asserting that the grounds surrounding this Asylum [when completed] will be second to none in the State for beauty of design or magnificence in scenery."[52] Dr. Clarke described the benefits of a beautiful landscape in terms of its curative function:

> The slope in front of the eastern division of the building,
> in which are the female wards, remains untouched and
> presents a forbidding appearance. It should be brought to
> harmonize with the gracefully finished lawn lying in front
> of the western division as early as practicable not only for

the purpose of pleasing the public eye, which it is always
well to do, but for stronger reasons, to present to the view
of those who look out for relief a landscape marked by
no violation of the laws of harmony. For surely no agency
contributes more potently to the relief of a mind disturbed
than strictly harmonious sensorial impressions.[53]

The asylum staff, the state of Ohio, and the village of Athens
embarked upon the experiment in moral treatment with confidence and hope placed in the curative nature of their methods.
Superintendent Holden contrasted the dawning of this new treatment with the methods of the early nineteenth century: "We no
longer meet the insane as we would a wild, ferocious animal, with
horror and fear, with handcuffs, chains and weapons for defense,
but we meet them as we meet other patients[,] with kind words;
words of sympathy and comfort, try to gain their confidence, teach
them you are their friend, and will do them no injury, and rarely
indeed will it be necessary to employ any means of restraint."[54]

The experiment was pursued vigorously for nearly twenty years.
Superintendents and staff worked hard to acquire clean water, prevent suicides, cope with political reorganization and the resultant
constant changing of staff, keep the building and furnishings in
good repair, balance the budget, and treat a staggering array of disorders and conditions with, in comparison to today's array of medications and treatment modalities, what were very limited means.
The asylum brought telephone and railroad service to Athens and
served as a huge market for its goods and services. Superintendent Richardson hired the first female asylum assistant physician in
America, Dr. Agnes Johnson of Zanesville, Ohio,[55] to improve the
care provided for women, and he also persuaded Ohio's legislature
to fund the first patient dining rooms at any American asylum,
so that rather than eating in their wards patients might be served
family-style in dining rooms with white tablecloths. Ultimately the
experiment ended, a casualty of both overcrowding and medical
progress. Richardson, who weathered Ohio's political spoils system to serve at Athens with national distinction from 1881 to 1890,
wrote of his discouragement about politics, overcrowding, and the
difficulty of caring for those with chronic severe mental illness as
well as the infirm elderly. At the end of the century, new models of
psychiatric care rendered asylums essentially custodial rather than
curative. Psychiatry was transforming itself from an administrative,

moral, and institution-based discipline to a medical specialty based on laboratory research and a new "cottage plan" design for residential treatment.

But the moral treatment pursued at Athens between 1874 and 1893 was the result of the blossoming of an American impulse to provide humane, expert care for those with mental illness. It yielded treatment modalities that flourish today as adjuncts to mental health treatment, now reconceived with new names such as restorative gardening, milieu therapy, art therapy, horticulture therapy, and humanistic psychology. The experiment at Athens, dedicated to moral treatment and founded on hope for curing mental illness, flourished for twenty years as a lively community of thousands of patients, dozens of attendants and workers, a small cadre of physicians, the people of the village of Athens, the families of patients, politicians in Columbus and Washington, social reformers, and a shared landscape of parkland and farms. Superintendent Richardson's closing words in one of his reports to the trustees reflect his thoughts on the twenty-year experiment in psychiatry:

> We have pursued the same general plan of treatment
> followed during previous years and outlined in former
> reports. I am well satisfied with the results. I believe,
> however, that there is still room for improvement in
> our treatment of insanity, and in the present methods
> of caring for the insane, and it is our aim to show
> in some direction every year a growth, and to make
> constantly honest efforts to improve upon the past,
> basing our actions always upon the broad grounds of
> common humanity and genuine sympathy for those in
> misfortune and helpless dependence. We are in no way
> circumscribed, but are ready to use any means that may
> enable us to better care for our responsible charge. . . .
> We have done what we could to make the Athens
> Asylum an institution of which you as well as the people
> of the State of Ohio need not be ashamed, and the
> mistakes which we have made have been mistakes in
> judgment alone.[56]

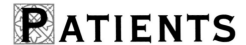ATIENTS

"Each Admission Represented a Poor, Helpless, Hopeless Sufferer"

On a cold day in the middle of winter, a little girl from Athens County became the Athens Lunatic Asylum's first patient. Her older brother accompanied her as, likely traveling by horse and wagon, they drove down the earthen road from town, across the Hockhocking River, and then up the great hill to the imposing Victorian structure. Eleven-year-old Alice had spent that Friday morning with her brother in commitment proceedings in the office of Athens County probate judge Leonidas Jewitt. Athens physician Dr. H. M. Lash and her brother provided witness and testimony as to her insanity.[1] After arriving at the asylum, they climbed its steps and entered the brick building—with its sixteen-foot ceilings, tile and marble floors, and oak woodwork— walked past the carpeted parlors ornamented with potted palms, and entered the west wing. There she was left by her brother with her clothing and little else.

Alice had a seizure disorder. Known at the time simply as epilepsy, seizure disorders were a great puzzle to American asylum physicians. Generally physicians resisted admitting patients with epilepsy, though by 1877 the Athens Asylum was caring, perhaps reluctantly, for patients with this diagnosis.[2] Superintendent Rutter in 1877 wrote to the hospital's trustees, "The hospital at this time contains forty (40) epileptics, all of whom are, by reason of their unfortunate complication, utterly unfit to be associated with any other class of patients."[3]

Effective treatment for epilepsy was not developed until the twentieth century, and nineteenth-century asylum physicians were at a loss in their efforts to care for patients with the disorder. Superintendent Holden of the Athens asylum in 1879 recommended to Ohio's governor a separate institution for Ohio's "epileptics," with the idea of isolating them so as not to disturb other patients. Holden noted: "This class of unfortunate beings should claim the attention of the State, and be provided for in a separate institution. The idea of their being associated with the insane is wrong. The fall, with the piercing cry of the epileptic, is shocking even to the sane person, but to those whose nervous constitutions are shattered, or about gone, it is excruciating and greatly detrimental. . . . [T]he epileptics are often dangerous and homicidal."[4]

When Alice arrived on January 16, 1874, her pulse and temperature were noted and a case file opened. The asylum physician who examined her described her as intelligent, kind, and cheerful. Her temperament was noted as "excitable" and her health apparently good. The admitting physician wrote that she "has swallowed pins and cut herself with glass as attempts at suicide. The attacks vary in duration and occur from two days or a week, at times more mild than at others. She appears to have warning of an approaching paroxysm."[5]

One can only imagine Alice's life as a young girl with a seizure disorder among three hundred or more women of all ages with a variety of mental illnesses. The medical notes documenting her progress describe the seizures and her recovery from them.

> 1/21[/74]: Had one paroxysm. Not very severe, stretched and tossed herself about in bed, jaws firmly closed. She did strike and scratch her nurse and remained partly conscious during the whole paroxysm. Was as well as usual the next morning except a slight soreness in muscles of limb and some headache.

> 1/27/74: Had slight paroxysm last night similar in form to preceding much shorter in duration and less recovery after. Symptoms are much the same as previous.

> 1/28/74: Had a mild attack at going to bed 8 pm, no symptoms remaining the following morning.

> 1/29/74: Had one other mild paroxysm last night, no remaining symptoms this morning.

> 2/15/74: Has had no attacks since the above date and is doing very well at present.[6]

The casebook does not note what became of Alice or how long she lived at the asylum. Genealogical records, though, suggest that she married in Michigan in 1879 and died in Los Angeles at the age of eighty in 1943.

The asylum accepted and cared for a diversity of patients. The elderly with dementia, women in need of care after childbirth, persons who had attempted suicide or harmed others, those committing crimes while mentally ill, persons with drug and alcohol addictions, and persons with what would be diagnosed today as schizophrenia, depression, or bipolar disorder are examples of the wide variety of the patients treated for conditions considered to be mental illness in late Victorian America.

Three documents were required to commit a person to an asylum in Ohio: a medical certificate from a physician certifying insanity; a request for commitment from the probate court with the names of witnesses; and a paper prepared by the asylum accepting the patient and noting the date, number assigned, age, and county of residence. Nearly a century's worth of these documents—many thousands of them—are archived with Ohio University Libraries. Folded, packed in letter-sized folios, layered with a fine sifting of dust accumulated over 135 years, and tied with faded red ribbons, the commitment papers reveal many details about asylum patients: age, health, family situation, symptoms, and the medical witness's best guess as to the cause of the bout of insanity.[7] Each of Ohio's eighty-eight counties had its own medical certificate and request for commitment; thus, the documents vary according to the originating county. The forms for each county evolved over time as to the kinds of details recorded. Some, filed away and undisturbed since 1874, display elaborate wax seals in still-brilliant golds and cadmium reds, and all bear the individual handwriting of physicians and probate judges with notes sometimes attached or written in the margins in ink or pencil. Officials wrote their notes with fountain pens and ink; one learns, as one reads through hundreds of these papers, to decipher the peculiarities of individual handwriting and the conventions of nineteenth-century penmanship. The documents contain the official legal and medical narratives of each of the 4,511 persons admitted between 1874 and 1893. Behind each official story couched in clinical language lie the struggles, pain, and sometimes the death of patients.[8] The narratives presented here are constructed from the stark facts offered in the medical evaluations; from the occasional departures from the measured clinical and judicial language in the commitment papers by officials explaining extraordinary medical events or pleading for swift action; and from notes and letters written by patients that were confiscated and preserved in files by asylum staff.

Two casebooks (one for men and one for women) maintained by asylum medical staff are kept under lock and key at the library of the Ohio Historical Society in Columbus, Ohio. Measuring eighteen inches tall by twelve inches wide, the casebooks, labeled with gold letters, are bound in oxblood leather and tan suede, with endpapers of marbled maroon, cream, teal, burgundy, royal blue, and yellow, and contain entries handwritten in ink on preprinted forms. Because the creamy white forms with light blue lines are printed on thick paper with a high cotton rag content, they are sturdy and beautifully preserved today, nearly 150 years later. The men's casebook is rich in details about the condition of patients at admission, though records cease in the spring of 1874 with Male Patient 179. Updates in the form of Progress of Case notes for these original 179 male patients were made every few months until mid-1875, at which time the effort was either abandoned or a new method of tracking patient progress (now lost to history) was in-stituted. One wonders whether by 1875, when the average daily number of patients stood at 597, the asylum's two assistant physi-cians were overwhelmed by the volume of work and simply ceased taking notes. The women's casebook contrasts with the men's. Details for female patients upon admission contain much less de-tail, and Progress of Case notes ceased altogether in January 1874, with the admission of the tenth female to the asylum.

Though the asylum was designed for only 572 patients, by 1876 the asylum's average daily count had reached 646. Superintendent Gundry advised the hospital's trustees in 1876 of crowded condi-tions: "One fact which these (statistical) tables will fail to show as vividly as your frequent visits to the Hospital during the past year must have impressed upon your consideration is the crowded condition of the Hospital. It is not yet three years since the first patient was admitted within these walls, and the wards are now over-crowded. There are more than seventy (70) patients in excess of the number this house was designed to accommodate."[9]

In 1886, the asylum's staff was caring for 672 patients each day, exceeding its intended capacity by a hundred patients. Even with the 1887 addition of space for 36 men and as many women, bringing the asylum's capacity to 644, in 1893 the asylum remained crowded, with an average daily occupancy of 813, or 169 patients over capacity.

When it opened, the asylum at Athens served twenty-eight of Ohio's eighty-eight counties. (Using today's mental health care language, the asylum's catchment area comprised twenty-eight counties in the rural south and southeast quadrant of Ohio.) State asylums in Columbus, Cincinnati, Cleveland, and Dayton served the rest of the state, and patients were sometimes sent from there to the asylum at Athens to relieve crowded wards. Athens received a hundred or more patients during the nineteenth century from sister institutions in Ohio; these patients arrived without case records and came usually in groups of a dozen or more, accompanied only by a list of their names, addresses, and age. Likely the patients transferring from Ohio's urban centers arrived by train, as transport by road to Athens was difficult in the nineteenth century, with axle-deep mud in the winter and spring making wagon and coach passage travel to the asylum nearly impossible at times.[10]

FIGURE 2.1 Service area of the Athens Lunatic Asylum in southeastern Ohio, 1874. *Originally published in* The New People's Universal Cyclopedia of Universal Knowledge *(New York: Phillips and Hunt, 1885).*

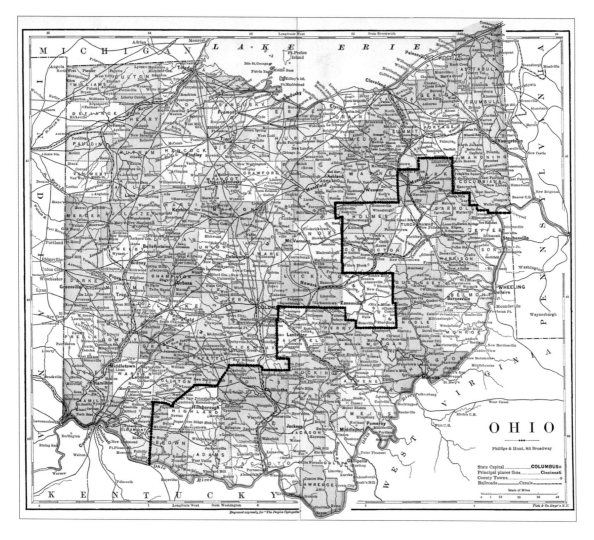

The asylum's commitment documents reveal that the admissions process dealt with every possible category of patient. Nineteenth-century mental illness diagnostic systems were based on the work of the French asylum physician Philippe Pinel.[11] Ohio asylum physicians practicing during the moral treatment era classified patients into eight categories: mania, mania with epilepsy, monomania (an obsession causing mental disarray), paresis (neurosyphilis eventually ending in dementia and death), melancholia (depression), five subcategories of dementia, imbecility, and finally not insane. These categories and the number of patients fitting each description were listed each year in the asylum's annual report.

Much more diverse were the causes ascribed to mental illness, their relationships to mental illness sometimes inscrutable.[12] Sixty-nine possible "physical" causes were tallied annually, including fevers, head and spinal injuries, sunstroke, apoplectic attack, dysentery, pneumonia and asthma, menstrual derangements, change of life, lactation, pregnancy, syphilis, masturbation,[13] intemperance, inhalation of nitrous oxide, lead poisoning, opium eating, bathing while overheated, excessive use of tobacco, exposure, loss of sight, and excessive heat. Twenty-seven possible "moral" causes were thought to underlie mental illness in the taxonomy of causation of nineteenth-century asylum medicine. Chief among them were business and financial troubles, domestic troubles, grief at loss of friends or family, and poverty and loss of money. Other moral causes tallied at Ohio's asylums each year were disappointment, fright, religious excitement, abuse by relatives, prison life, slander, spiritualism, attempted rape, unmarried life, and repression by parents. Community physicians speculated about an even broader array of causation as they filled out patients' commitment papers, including reasons such as fording a cold creek while menstruating, uterine troubles, typhoid fever, cannonading, the shock of enduring a great storm at sea while immigrating to America from Germany, physical prostration from overexertion, unwise disposition of property, hard drinking, and disease of the stomach and bowel. The accounts of the lives of the patients in this chapter are based on the observations and descriptions of community physicians and probate judges, surviving case notes from asylum physicians, testimony and descriptions from family and friends, and in some instances the writings of patients themselves.

Male Patient 1, a merchant from an eastern Ohio county bordering the Ohio River, was admitted to the asylum on Sunday, January 11, 1874. The case notes relate that he was sixty-two years old, married, Methodist, and possessed of a "good education." His parents had immigrated to America from Ireland and died before his admission. In describing the patient's disposition and health, the admitting asylum physician noted that he was a quick-tempered, kind, sober, and industrious man with light brown hair. Depressed and in poor health for three months, he feared financial ruin. He had good reason to be worried about his business: at that time, Americans were living through the Long Depression. We learn that the "exciting cause of his mental illness" was judged to be "business perplexity and general ill health" and that he was depressed "respecting his future condition and fear of pecuniary loss." By the time of admission, he was weak in body with "paroxysmal attacks of jumping and noise," had made an attempt to hang himself, and was thought to be dangerous and "apt to strike people suddenly." He had lucid moments in which his mind functioned well, but at other times he was "sometimes excited and tries to fight and bite." He slept poorly. We learn that his "vegetative functioning" was poor, he possessed a craving appetite, his bowels were constipated, his eyes were blue, his vision was good, and his hearing, smell, and taste were unremarkable. Six entries describing his condition appear in the casebook:

January 11: 98 1/2 temperature, pulse 64, weight 100 pounds. Strength 60 on the Dynamometer.[14] Feeling almost normal. Seems to be much better and in good spirits.

January 20: temperature 98 1/4, pulse 64, weight 102 pounds. Seems to be some better. Had a bad day on the 18th, confined mostly to the forenoon and was about as bad as when brought here.

February 7: Pulse 60, strength 70, weight 104 pounds. Improving slowly. Does not have those spells of mania as when he came except some and then not so bad.

May 2: About the same as when first admitted mentally but much stronger physically. Tried to but [*sic*] his head against the wall about a week ago.

May 8: Has become jaundiced in the conjunctival some and in the skin a little.

May 16: Still continues considerably yellow. Was given a pill containing 1/2 gr. Potassium & 1 gr. Aloes.

May 17: Has taken meat within the last 18 hours. Remains
   weak and is rather drowsy most of the time.

May 28: Taken away (by his brother who was a physician).[15]

The last entry notes that Male Patient 1 died at home six weeks later.

The asylum records contain many other instances of men, especially older men, hospitalized for depression and worry surrounding financial circumstances. Male Patient 150, a sixty-year-old farmer, is another example. He entered the asylum for an illness "one year of duration, the exciting cause of which is Financial Embarassment." Some remained preoccupied with finances while in the asylum, writing for money to purchase clothes or as repayment of debt. Families of men who were depressed, violent, and out of work brought them to the asylum as a last resort. A thirty-year-old man from Chillicothe was hospitalized with "melancholia with incipient dementia (caused by) failure in business."[16] A sixty-year-old man was hospitalized after having been "thrown out of employment" and having attempted "violence upon himself and others."[17] A farmer, age twenty-six and married, fell into a depression after the death of his father, complicated by financial worries and his responsibilities as executor of his father's estate. The medical witness described the history of his case as "one month, for the first two weeks slight mental disturbance followed by violent fits of insanity. The cause is depression of mind from the recent death of his father, of whom he is Executor and anxiety relative to pecuniary matters." The physician and the asylum also cited a "blow to the head" occasioned by a fall and injury to the right side of the head. The young farmer remained hospitalized at the asylum for a month, after which he was sent home "seemingly almost well." Presumably the asylum's regimen of rest and purposeful activity was more curative than the home treatment he received: "blistering the nape of the neck."[18] A fifty-year-old farmer from the Ohio River town of Portsmouth was committed by his wife in 1874 because he had attempted suicide by shooting himself. This man had been hospitalized twenty years earlier at the asylum in Columbus, Ohio, but was at home on his farm in 1874 when he attempted suicide.[19] During the previous three weeks, he had "acted strangely, avoiding the society of friends and imagines there are men on the roof of his own house and sometimes that of his neighbors." The medical witness and the asylum's admission notes describe him as a man "with all sorts of delusions about his wife and children being in the fires at

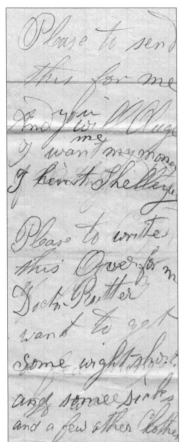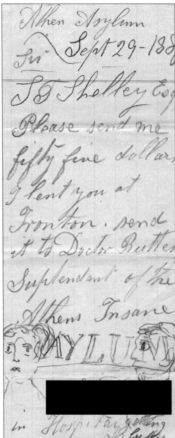

FIGURE 2.2 Letter and note from patient, 1880. *Courtesy of the Mahn Center for Archives and Special Collections, Ohio University Libraries.*

the boilerhouse" and who "sometimes imagines he is being robbed at night and goes about the house naked." Hospitalized in February 1874, he arrived "at times very much depressed and thinks all his friends have deserted him." Three months later he was "still very much discontented with being kept here," and though his general health was good, he "did not eat much." In July 1874, his condition was much the same. The casebook records that in July he "got outside one day and ran to the hill but did not attempt to go farther." In September, he was taken home by his family.[20]

The new asylum provided a place for southern Ohio's poorhouses (also known as county homes or infirmaries) to relocate their residents thought to be mentally ill.[21] Among the first patients admitted to the asylum at Athens were four women from the Ross County Home: Female Patients 3, 4, 5, and 6. Their cases for insanity, brought before the probate court in Chillicothe on the afternoon of January 16, 1874, had been prepared that morning by the physician attending the county home. The court determined that the women were unable to attend the probate hearing in the judge's chambers, and they were represented, with no other witnesses, by the physician attending the county home. At the proceedings, they were all found to be insane and eligible for commitment to a state asylum. Two days later, the four women, one of them in a straitjacket, traveled together to Athens (accompanied by the Ross County sheriff) and were admitted to the asylum on January 19. The reports of the medical witness and the asylum casebook provide a glimpse into the lives and conditions of these four women from the poorhouse.

Female Patient 3, age thirty-two, was determined to have been mentally ill for five years. The physician serving as medical witness summarized the grim facts of her condition: "The cause of her illness is exposure after confinement (childbirth) with her last child, want, and a brutal husband. She appeared entirely recovered at the end of her first year (at the Infirmary) and was sent home but relapsed. Medical treatment has consisted of nourishing food and cold baths."[22]

Female Patient 4, a forty-year-old widow, traveled to the asylum wearing "sleeves," the Victorian name for a straitjacket. The physician determined that she had been insane for five years and wrote only of her history, "Cause unknown—was in Asylum at Columbus Ohio for three years past, then confined in the County Infirmary." From the casebook we learn that she "was brought in sleeves by sheriff," that she had been treated previously at the Central Asylum at Columbus for "paroxysms of excitement," and that her health was "tolerable good" but her sight and hearing were failing. The casebook holds one note about her progress, written a few weeks later on February 2, 1874: "[She] remains much the same as when admitted—general health tolerable good, at times violent, destructive and dangerous."

The medical witness physician made one note in regard to Female Patient 5, who was thirty-eight: "I found her at the Infirmary five years ago, insane—she has failed in her speech and articulation, in the last six months very much. The cause is unknown except her father was a drunkard and abusive. There have been no attempts of violence." An asylum physician noted a few weeks after her admission that she "remains the same as when admitted both physically and mentally. She is very noisy at times."[23]

We learn from the Ross County certificate of insanity that Female Patient 6 was age fifty-nine and "she has been insane for over five years—was in Asylum at Columbus two years and the last time in the infirmary. Cause: unhappy family relations with her husband." After she was admitted to the asylum at Athens, one case note was entered for her, on February 2, 1874: "Failing sight and deficient hearing. [She] has not improved since her admission into the Asylum. She is very excitable at times."

Difficulty following childbirth—exhaustion, depression, illness, lack of proper care—brought many women to the asylum. Ill with mastitis and depressed following the birth of her third child, the wife of a Civil War veteran was hospitalized in 1874 by her doctor and her husband, becoming Female Patient 36.[24] Her doctor wrote,

> Duration of her illness is about six months, the exciting cause of which is probably childbirth or the puerperal state.[25] [She] has attempted violence upon herself. She has taken remedies to quiet her nervous system, such as Chloral Bromides and Morphine, but not regularly nor in large enough doses to have much effect. . . . About three months after confinement and while suffering with repeated mammary abscesses & much pain & loss of sleep she first began to exhibit symptoms of Insanity[.] [S]he has been very melancholy—has several times attempted suicide & says she is fearful she may kill her child. Does not eat or sleep enough[;] requires constant watching.

The casebook noted that she had been brought by her husband to the asylum suffering from an abscess of both breasts and talking of suicide by hanging, poison, or drowning. She recovered and returned home, and a few years later she visited Boston and wrote a memoir of her visit there to Henry Wadsworth Longfellow's garden, where he presented her with a rose. The son whose birth precipitated her illness went on to work for the Internal Revenue Service and lived to the age of eighty-one.

Another mother and her child did not fare so well. A probate judge in Zanesville, Ohio, added this note to the asylum superintendent to the standard commitment form for Female Patient 62, emphasizing the desperate situation of his charge, an unmarried woman who had killed her child:

> March 3, 1874
> Dr. R. Gundry:
>   Athens, O.
>
> Dear Sir:
>   In the case of _____, I copy the following from the Medical Certificate. The exciting cause of her Insanity "is

trouble growing out of a bastard child. She murdered her child with an ax and does not attempt to conceal it. She has been worse during her menstrual period. She imagines spirits present and talking with her."

Any information that I can give you regarding any of the patients sent from here will be cheerfully given.

Very Respectfully
L. R. Landfear
Probate Judge

Commitment for insanity in circumstances of unwed motherhood was not unheard of. Female Patient 192, a twenty-eight-year-old woman from Zanesville, Ohio, was hospitalized ostensibly for guilt over having disgraced her family in this manner. Explained the medical witness,

The exciting cause of disease: compunction for having disgraced herself and family. Has not attempted violence. Her mind was devoted as much as possible by all who knew her. Chloral & bromide & Potassia were given to procure sleep, other remidees we used as tonics etc. . . . I would say there are other circumstances which would have tendency to throw further light upon the subject. Last Spring she had an Illegitimate child, and from that time never left the house. During Aug. and Sept. she nursed a Sister who had Typhoid Fever and during that time the first symptoms of Insanity were detected.

Women were also declared insane because of the strain of bearing many children. A twenty-six-year-old mother from the Columbus area was sent to the Athens asylum because of "over-anxiety about her children. The primary cause is over-child bearing, having had five children in six years." Her doctor suggested that she might be soon cured at the asylum and could perhaps "make a rappid recovery if she can have proper care, treatment and rest."[26]

In Victorian America, sexually transmitted disease, especially syphilis, was of medical, moral, and social concern. In part because of the association of the disease with prostitution, women were thought to be responsible for spreading the disease and were urged to keep themselves clean. A medical treatise on the treatment of syphilis from 1842 notes, "If, in general, women were more cleanly and careful of themselves, the venereal disease would be far less common."[27]

Both women and men were encouraged by their physicians not to marry if they had syphilis, to prevent spreading the disease.

Female Patient 277, a new bride twenty years of age, had contracted syphilis while visiting Wheeling, West Virginia, when she was nineteen.[28] She visited a doctor in Mount Vernon, Ohio, and he treated her, though he urged her not to follow through with plans to marry. Despite this advice, marry she did. Following the wedding, she and her husband visited another physician regarded as a "quack" by her Mount Vernon physician. The "quack," without examining her, told her she was pregnant and infected with syphilis and sent her back to her father's home. Here unfolded a drama involving suicide attempts, which led to her commitment to the asylum at Athens on June 5, 1874.[29] Her Mount Vernon physician prepared her commitment papers with no mention of syphilis, saving that for a private letter to the asylum superintendent.

> Statement of Medical Witness to the Probate Court:
> I hereby certify that I have examined Mrs. _____, State of Ohio and find her insane. I believe her now to be free from any infectious disease or vermin.
> She is twenty years of age. On Wednesday May 28th 1874 I was called upon to see the aforesaid lady found her at the Commercial House in Mt. Vernon, Ohio in bed[.] [H]er voice was husky, pupils contracted, she acknowledged to having taken morphine with a view of destroying her life[:] under a threat from me that her trunk should be examined she gave me a bottle containing 10 1/2 grains of Sulphate of Morphine. Strong Coffee was ordered and a close watch kept. On Thursday evening following upon hearing her Father's voice, she shot herself in the thorax, the ball entered at the middle and near the left side of the Sternum, and passed in an outward direction and now lies in the soft parts covering the left side of the Thorax. None of the parties were ever in an Asylum. Mrs. _____ has never had Epilepsy. This person has made two attempts to take her life, and of which I have knowledge. The treatment has been good nutritious diet and a sedative. She now says that she does not want to recover, has attempted to probe the wound with her fingers.

Her physician attached a letter describing the year-long unfolding of the situation, which included the diagnosis of syphilis and follow-up treatment by the "quack," details that he wished to spare the patient's parents. His notes, down to the blue silk dress purchased by the bride, give an unusually vivid picture of the difficulties of this young woman.

June 1st, 1874
To the Superintendent of the Lunatic Asylum at Athens, Ohio

Dear doctor,

I take this opportunity to give you some more information in regard to _____ than I felt called upon to make in the Certificate. I write you expecting that what I now reveal will be kept a secret for the sake of the father and mother of this unfortunate woman. She first consulted me for a private disease about the middle of last January. Said she contracted it 2 months prior in Wheeling Va. I made an examination and found a chancre and multiple bubers in both groins. I regarded the case one of true Syphilis and so treated it. In a few weeks she had sore throat & an eruption. Under the use of Hyd. Bichloride & Tinct. Ferri internally and applications of nitrate of silver the chancre healed, eruptions & sore throat disappeared. She remained under my care 2 1/2 months when I regarded her cured. She told me that she was engaged to be married, time had been set—I told her the danger of getting married in that condition and advised her to postpone the day indefinitely[.] [T]his she said [she] could not do and was married since [that] time in April[.] [O]n her way to the home of her husband they stopped in Zanesville and consulted a quack doctor by the name of _____. Without any vaginal examination he pronounced her badly diseased and pregnant—and sent her back to her father. On Wednesday May 20th she started from her father's with the view of joining her husband. She stopped in Zanesville and consulted the Quack[;] prior to leaving home she tried to poison herself with strychnine. She purchased in Zanesville a beautiful blue silk dress, with kid slippers and other articles of dress to match and returned to this city on Saturday May 23rd. She came to my office (after an absence of some 8 weeks). I made an examination and could not find any evidence of disease. Tried hard to satisfy her . . . and told her to seek the advice of some regular physician. She took that . . . advice and again chose a quack. After this she proceeded at once to the carrying out of her plan. First on Tuesday at 10 and 10 1/2 PM and [again] Wednesday 4 AM she took a dose of morphine in all 45 grains. I saw her on Wednesday 11 AM, found her pupils contracted, voice husky, said she had vomited after each dose. Under threat that her trunk should be examined she gave me up what Morphine she had left & said she would go on with her husband. Her father came before she got started and the moment she heard his voice she shot herself. . . . The cause of her insanity is very plain I think. I expect that under your professional care & skill she will be returned entirely cured both in body and mind.

    Yours,
      _____, MD

The new bride entered the asylum at Athens four days later on June 5 as Female Patient 277.

In 1874, another bride was found to be insane and was hospitalized with witness provided by two female friends. Distraught that she had married the wrong man, Female Patient 242 was suicidal and had to be watched constantly by friends. The physician explained, "The exciting cause is as I learn Matrimonial disappointment. She is sane on some subjects and has perfect lucid intervals in which she is sane on all. She has attempted violence upon herself. I am of [the] opinion that if confined for a few weeks under kind treatment, that she will entirely recover as suicide is her only Mania." The probate judge added a separate letter explaining the situation to the superintendent:

Dr. Gundry

Dear Sir:
    Inclosed please find papers in case of _____[,] a married lady[;] it appears that she is sensible of having disappointed someone else by Marrying her present husband and for that reason she ought to put herself out of the way of all. She finds no fault with her husband[.] She has repeatedly attempted Suicide by different means. Her friends are compelled to guard her continually, she seems to be reasonable in other matters. Please reply at

your earliest convenience, as she is being kept here to wait the reply.

> Respectfully etc.
> J. C. Evans
> PJ [Probate Judge]

The sights, sounds, and injuries of the battlefields of the American Civil War induced trauma and illness that, for some, resulted in commitment to the asylum. Male Patient 216, from a farm along the Ohio River, was hospitalized because of a mental illness dating from 1865. His physician wrote that the cause of his illness was "Typhoid fever, from which he suffered while in the Army during the year of 1864. [He] has made attempts of violence upon his family and others." This veteran had been a private in the 91st Regiment of the Ohio Infantry. Before his illness, he participated in the West Virginia war theater, including a raid up the Kanawha River and pursuit of Morgan's Raiders.

Male Patient 231, a private in the 188th Ohio Infantry, was admitted to the Athens asylum in 1874 following ten years of mental illness attributed to the trauma of the sounds of battle. His physician describes his case, which dated from 1864, as a "case of chronic mania, he was in an asylum about five years ago. The cause is nervous derangement, probably acquired while in the Army. He received a sudden shock from cannonading."

Male Patient 3 enlisted in the Ohio 77th Infantry Regiment at the age of fifteen and endured near-constant battle conditions until the war's end, when he had his first "attack" of mental illness. The medical report committing him in 1874 noted, "About seven years ago [he] had an attack lasting two or three months, has had three or four attacks since. He has made threats of violence upon himself and also upon others." The teenager fought with his regiment in the spring of 1862 at Shiloh, the bloodiest battle in U.S. history at that time. Descriptions of the battlefield at Shiloh note the corpse-littered ground, creating a deadly psychological effect. The young soldier pressed on with his unit to the siege of Corinth, then to Chickamauga, and finally to the siege of Atlanta before falling psychologically ill.

Some Civil War veterans were sent to asylums because their violent behavior could not be controlled at home. Male Patient 243, a private in the Ohio Infantry, was hospitalized at Athens in 1874, according to the medical witness because of a blow on the head received while in the U.S. Army in 1863, when he was fifteen years old. He was soon hospitalized in the state asylum at Columbus, Ohio, which burned in 1868, no doubt creating further trauma for this veteran. Since then he had been confined at home, in Marietta, Ohio, "subject to paroxysms of violent mania." His father initiated his second hospitalization when the Athens asylum opened in 1874.

Families of soldiers who were killed suffered as well. Some were unable to recover and required hospitalization. An Ohio mother, age sixty-four, remained stricken with grief over the death of her son in the war, and her family brought her for commitment to the asylum, where she became Female Patient 286. The medical witness noted,

> This is to certify that I have this day examined Mrs. _____, a Widow Lady about 64 years of age, and find her labouring under that species of Insanity known by the name of Monia Mania, arriseing from the distress caused by her son, being killed in the late War[.] [S]he has been three times to the Asylum, and discharged each time cured[;] she has been home from the Asylum this last time two years and four months, continued Well and undisturbed in her mind until the first day of Last March, when she began to show symptoms of mental aberration— Since which time she has been more or less noisy and troublesome, being more so whenever the subject matter of her son is brought to her mind[.] [T]he Physical health is good, [and she] has been under no medical treatment, I therefore feel confident that removal to some asylum where she can get a proper Treatment will soon restore her Mind.

Another mother, Female Patient 749, was hospitalized in 1874 because of "grief of the death of her son in the Army."

Male Patient 819, age twenty-eight, was admitted to the asylum by way of special legislation passed by the Ohio General Assembly. He had been sent to Athens from his family home in Philadelphia to live with an uncle. Because he was not a resident of Ohio, an act of the Ohio General Assembly was required for his admission to the asylum. His admission papers consist of a small certificate with a two-and-a-half-inch red wax seal signed by the Ohio secretary of state. Once in the asylum, he penned a series of plaintive notes to family members and to asylum physicians asking for help in going home. Written in purple ink, some in English and others in German, the letters were never sent but kept instead in asylum files. The undated letters repeatedly inquire about coming home; one letter directs his uncle in Athens to send him a drum over at the asylum.

To Emil S., N. 6th Street Philadelphia

Dear brother Emil
    I am wanting to wait to get home. I will inform you how I am getting along which to let you know about my coming home, since 10 years away from home . . . telegraph immediately and want to know whether farther is well nothing more at present hoping to see you soon.

Leon S.
Atlanta

Dear brother Leon S.
    I would like to know how soon you will be in Philadelphia or you could send me a telegraph that you are well about my traveling home myself alone I was going to ask you about coming home telegraph to send me home.
    This is all at present

Solomon S.
Marshall, Missouri

Dear brother Solomon,
    Hoping to see you soon I will let you know how soon. I will be at home and hoping that you are well and all I which to now [*sic*] whether you are going home. This it would be better at home so good bye at present.
    Nothing more.

Mr. Abraham _____.
Please Telegraph to Mr. Isaac _____. to bring his son home.

Mr. Abraham S., Athens
Bring over one drum at for _____.

Mr. Abraham S.
Please send over one drum for _____.

Dr. Rutter
Dr. Kelly

Dr. Rutter & Dr. Kelly
    Please leave me know whether I can
leave after dinner for my home my farther
will pay for the time that I stayed in Athens
and what it cost my farther will pay what it
cost to travel home to Philadelphia.[30]

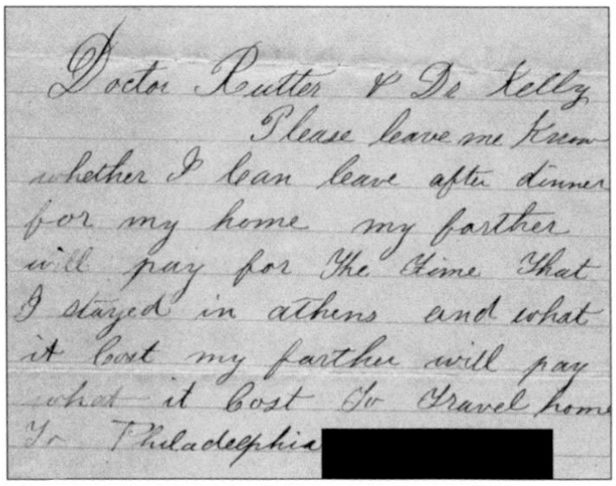

FIGURE 2.3
Note from Male
Patient 819 to
Superintendent
Rutter and Dr.
Kelly, 1880. *Courtesy
of the Mahn Center for
Archives and Special
Collections, Ohio
University Libraries.*

Some patients resisted hospitalization by taking matters into
their own hands and escaping or making plans to leave.[31] Their
strong feelings and inventive plans are recorded in their own letters as well as in the asylum's casebook. Male Patient 1060, a Captain C. of the Ohio River town of Marietta,[32] was hospitalized by
family and friends, who inquired by letter as to his well-being.

    Marietta, Ohio July 8, 1880.
    The Surgeon In Charge of the Asylum Athens O.

    Dear Sir
        Will you please keep us informed of Capt. C. and
    how he is getting along and what prospects there is of
    his recovery. His sister sent his clothes but did not here
    whether he rec'd them hope he did, please give us your
    Opinion and oblige.

        Yours Respectfully,
        Capt. Ben F. Hall[33]

Captain C., meanwhile, was making plans to escape from the asylum, which he documented in a note written in pencil on a scrap
of paper that was confiscated and filed by asylum staff.

To John Smart:

Friend John, as I have become convinced that my imprisonment has turned into persecution you are all I have left to depend on now I want you to go and hunt up a saw blade new or old it will be better if fine and hand it up to me at the third windo from the angle don't fail to get me something this evening for I want to start for home to night also get me a good stout heavy club to defend myself with don't fail me in the name of the God we both serve and worship. I will be waiting for you.[34]

He did not escape; he died there two years later and was buried in the asylum cemetery, where his remains rest today.

Male Patient 38, a thirty-three-year-old unmarried railroad engineer from the Columbus area, was admitted to the Athens asylum on the testimony of a medical witness stating that "the patient is harmless and the attack of insanity is mild consisting mainly of misinterpretation." He escaped after two months of hospitalization, taking another patient with him, by cutting open his door with a chisel left in the ward by a carpenter. Two months later he returned of his own accord, only to escape again, "going west on the 10:30 a.m. train." He again returned and made his final escape on July 24 by picking the lock on his door.

Male Patient 176, an unmarried twenty-five-year-old man from Columbus, was sentenced to the state penitentiary for theft; soon after, he had an "attack of insanity" and was moved to the Athens asylum, and the cause of his insanity was assessed at admission as intemperance. The next day his condition was recorded: "[A]fter getting over his drunk spell has appeared to be perfectly sane." Two weeks later, he "became drunk from whiskey which he got in some mysterious way."[35] Within a month he departed; the casebook notes, "Escaped last night by breaking out one of the bars in the iron sash. In the evening he had stolen $64 in money from an attendant and $6000 in notes. All this he took with him."

Women and men alike might be sent to the asylum because family and community considered them dangerous. Male Patient 209, a fifteen-year-old boy, was hospitalized following the death of his father: "For six months he has been taken with frequent mad fits and becomes enraged and threatens to kill some of his folks and himself. Cause: mental trouble from the death of his Father some seven months since, and I suspicion onanisme." A young farmer, age twenty-eight, was hospitalized for fear that he would kill his family and take his own life. Wrote the medical witness, "He has for some time carried a revolver, razor, and sling shot. Swears he will kill all the family and any one else he can get his hands on. Has threatened to kill his wife on several occasions. Was going to kill his wife and then himself. He is violent at times, and destructive."[36]

Thirty-nine-year-old Male Patient 922, from Zanesville, Ohio, was hospitalized because he "has for some time imagined himself possessed of great powers and has abused his wife . . . and has made attempts of violence upon others . . . he being at large is very dangerous to the community." While in the asylum, he wrote letters to family and friends, sometimes using the pen names of Rat Trap Man and The Bone Man. He was moved to express himself in verse, including an ode that reflects on the comfort and virtues of family (figure 2.4).

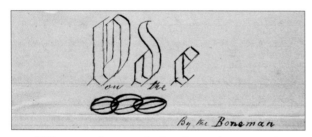

FIGURE 2.4
Letter from patient.
Courtesy of the Mahn Center for Archives and Special Collections, Ohio University Libraries.

When you know, of a brother, who is much in need,
And know, that *comfort,* is to him a Blendship,
Than take him in, and comfort him, indeed;
And he shurely *will than say; this is,* Friendship.

When a better half, you seek for a wife
Be shure, that she is virtuos, as Angels, above.
A virtuos woman, is the only jewel in a man's life.
Especially *when true and pure, in regard* to Love.

Then when you hear the sweet names, my dear brother,
My dear father, my dear Husband, you are so good
Remember your Parent, especially your dear mother
When in your boyhood, she explained to you
The Meaning of Friendship, Love & Truth.

The following ode appears to reflect on a judge whose "knowledge of law is the worse I ever saw."

Ode on 2 Squires, with the name of
    Buck
One from Xenia, the other from New Lexington O.

Squire "Buck" you are a little "off"—
At best *you* are N. G.
Your knowledge ? Law! _ & _
    Is the worse, I ever saw,
And a "bock" you ever will be.

I once saw a Sawbock
    Which was at the time on a draw
And just as the saw, was on _____ made go
So your tongue wags to and fro
    When displaying knowledge of Law.

Now this man Buck, is a genuine bugger
    Very likely an old Kentucker
    When to him a case is brought before
    The defendant, He'll surely bind him o'er
So natural does a sucker.

Other patients expressed themselves by carving marks into the stone ledges of the windows of their rooms (figure 2.5).

Fifty-seven-year-old Male Patient 24 had been ill and unmanageable by his family for twelve years. Hospitalized during the years

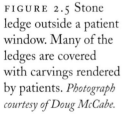

FIGURE 2.5 Stone ledge outside a patient window. Many of the ledges are covered with carvings rendered by patients. *Photograph courtesy of Doug McCabe.*

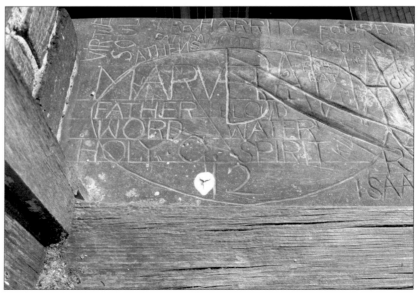

1861–66 in Columbus, he escaped and came home. When the Athens asylum opened, his family enlisted the support of a physician and had him committed again. Wrote his physician, "He labors at present under religious delusions, with acute mania. Talks incoherently, is violent, and unmanageable. Twelve years duration. He was first sent to an Asylum in 1861, remaining about five years when he escaped. Has frequently made threats of killing, commanded by the Lord to do so."

A longtime school superintendent, Male Patient 1988, was hospitalized by his friends because they feared he was homicidal. Divorced and living alone, he was committed after a two-month bout with depression. Noted his physician, "He can recollect nothing of any consequence and sleeps but very little. Concealed a hatchet under his bed, limited appetite, and slightly homicidal."

Male Patient 221, from Chillicothe, was hospitalized because he committed a murder and was found guilty by a jury because of insanity. Diagnosed with melancholia with incipient dementia caused by failure in business, he was determined by the medical witness to have been insane for four and a half years. A three-page handwritten document entitled "Inquest of Lunacy: Indictment for Murder in First Degree" described the process and at the end summarized the decision: "[W]e the jury do find that _____ is not now sane."

Women were likewise committed to the asylum because of violent or unruly behavior. The commitment records contain many accounts of women considered dangerous to themselves or others and committed. Female Patient 18 "threatened violence on herself & others. I am unable to state the medical treatment which has been pursued in her case; she has been subject to menstrual irregularities, and to some recent religious excitement. The condition is one of acute mania with quick pulse, insomnia and paroxysms of ungovernable excitement. Residence in an Asylum would probably effect a speedy improvement in her case." Female Patient 31, age thirty-one, had "recently attempted violence on members of her family and threatens to take her own life." And Female Patient 311, age forty-seven, had "been melancholic since the first of May 1874 and with acute mania a part of the time to this date. Duration: 3 months. Cause: originated in the year 1858 from suspension of menstruation but she has had three children since. Has made threats of violence upon others and Neighbors. Threats to burn property."

Parents who could not care for their mentally ill children also sought help from the local probate judge. A young man's uncle obtained commitment for his nephew on behalf of the young man's widowed mother, who was unable to care for him. Because the young man was no longer a resident of Ohio, the probate judge arranged for an act of the Ohio legislature to commit him to the asylum at Athens. It read, in part, "Where as _____, age thirty years unmarried was born in Gallipolis Gallia County and resided there with his parents until near manhood, when he went from home to provide for himself and whereas, after an absence of some twelve years he returns to the house of his widowed mother insane."[37] Male Patient 209, a fifteen-year-old boy mad with grief at the death of his father, was hospitalized because he was dangerous to himself and the rest of the family. The medical witness stated, "For six months he has been taken with frequent mad fits and becomes enraged and threatens to kill some of his folks and himself. The cause is mental trouble from the death of his father some seven months since."

Families brought relatives with delusions to probate court for commitment hearings. A sixty-one-year-old widow, Female Patient 1241, was hospitalized by her only child for delusions: "She imagines she sees the devil and witches. Talks about money all the time. Imagines hearing people talking about money." A thirty-one-year-old schoolteacher with a "good natural disposition," Male Patient 1912 was hospitalized because he "imagines he is being persecuted and that some one is giving him medicine in his coffee and that some one is trying to ruin him, and that everyone is against him." Female Patient 345, a quiet older woman living along the Ohio River, was hospitalized on the word of five community members who brought her before the probate court with the following information: "Mrs. _____ is quiet, lives alone, doing her own work, though quite infirm. Talks coherently but sometimes refers to visual hallucinations or certain insane delusions as to her bodily ailments that become matters of belief and indicate a disordered mind. Duration of insanity: 16 years." And Female Patient 331, age thirty, was declared insane because for ten days she imagined communications and directives from Christ. Her certificate of insanity reads, "She imagines that she has direct communications with our Saviour. That she can do nothing unless he tells her to do it. That she holds frequent conversations with Christ. Imagines that different members of family and friends are murdered. Has not attempted violence on herself or others. . . . [T]he probable cause of her insanity is menstrual derangement."

Adult family members who became too difficult for family and community to care for were also hospitalized. A fifty-five-year-old man, Male Patient 10, described as "intemperate in his habits" (he drank) suffered a loss of property followed by the death of his wife; he became unmanageable by family and friends. Wrote the medical witness, "Duration of insanity one year the exciting of which from loss of property, intemperance and in January last his wife died—since then he has grown gradually worse, and he now is wild. I learn that the man has been intemperate in his habits, but trouble as above indicated appears to have unbalanced his mind." A farmer was taken by his son to the asylum at Athens the month that it opened, making the fifty-mile journey from Morgan County in the dead of winter. The medical witness speculated that his illness stemmed from the death of one of his sons, and clearly his behavior had become too much for his family to manage. The asylum casebook records that this man, a Civil War veteran, was "despondent. Fears that someone is going to carry him off and drown or burn him. He is suicidal [and] has attempted once to cut his throat and hang himself. Tries to run off. Has an abdominal hernia caused by cutting his entrails out with a knife in an attempt to commit suicide." Several months later at the asylum, he was "still very melancholic at times. Thinks his friends have forgotten him and that someone is laying a mine beneath the floor which is to blow him up." By June he had been taken home by his son, though the asylum physicians judged that he was "not entirely well."[38] Women thought to be dangerous were also committed by their families, as in the case of the thirty-eight-year-old woman committed by her husband and brought to the asylum by a sheriff because she was noisy, excited, and had attempted to cut her husband's throat.[39]

A tendency to wander and roam was thought to be a symptom of insanity, and women prone to do so were hospitalized. The medical witness for Female Patient 33, age forty-four, wrote, "Duration of the disease is as nearly as can be ascertained of many years duration. No attempts to commit violence. The medical treatment pursued in the case has not been known. This is a mild case of long standing, manifested by great fickleness of purpose[,] occasional violent and causeless fits of passion, and a disposition to wander about." The medical certificate of insanity for twenty-five-year-old Female Patient 260 states, "All that is known is the general fact that she runs away in cold amidst brush and stones. It is her habit to run away from all attempts to examine into her condition and persistently refuse to take proposed remedies. Have been called to give testimony in this case with very slight means of determining many important questions; hence the certificate is of little practical value, except in a legal sense." And this forty-five-year-old woman became Female Patient 330 for wandering and talking about venereal disease: "She imagines that she is afflicted with Venereal diseases, and has made application for treatment to the various Physicians. She roams over the Country and relates her condition to persons generally."

The asylum accepted patients whose illness was ascribed to drug and alcohol use. Male Patient 341, a thirty-three-year-old farmer, was hospitalized for mental illness of one year's duration, "the existence of which is protracted use of alcoholic liquor." A twenty-eight-year-old physician was hospitalized by his father for drug use. Wrote his physician, "Has formed the cocaine habit. His actions are entirely at variance with mental soundness. There is great danger of his doing violence, both to himself and those about him. Supposed cause: *The excessive use of cocaine.*"[40] And a thirty-eight-year-old postmaster was hospitalized by his father-in-law, the county sheriff. Noted his physician, "Hallucinations and etc. caused by alcohol. Supposed cause: excess of alcoholic stimulant."[41]

Some patients died soon after admission, having arrived in a state of advanced physical illness. Superintendents of the asylum began to worry in their annual reports about the problem of families waiting too long to bring patients, so that they arrived in a "greatly debilitated condition." Female Patient 17, a native of Gallia County on the Ohio River, was sixty years old and had been hospitalized after an illness of two weeks' duration. Her medical witness wrote that "about two weeks ago she commenced screaming and hollering." Brought by the sheriff to the asylum in early February 1874, she was diagnosed with dementia. Obviously ill, she was monitored and her condition noted in the casebook each day from February 7 to February 9, when she died. By her third day at the asylum, her temperature had risen from 98 to 100 and her pulse was 120. The case notes made throughout the day and evening of February 9 suggest that one of the two assistant physicians had kept constant vigil at his patient's bedside all day and into the night until her death.

> She is getting very feeble [and] has a very bad cough with copious expectora.

Takes but little nourishment—growing weaker and refuses nourishment.

Remains very much the same.

Died at 11 o'clock PM. Apparently without any agony—been present at her bedside.[42]

Male Patient 12 died about five months after he was admitted, at age fifty-two. A shoemaker by trade, this man was born in Virginia and had been a resident of the Ohio River town of Gallipolis. The evidence of his insanity presented by the medical witness was that "about one year ago he became absent minded." We learn from the casebook that he had little education, was married, had brown hair that was "slightly greyed," hazel eyes, a "full bounding pulse," and was flabby. He was "not good in legs, could not feel unless pinched very hard." The admitting physician noted that "a considerable time between when a question is put to him and the answer received not very good. Forgot his children's names[,] said all the boys names were George. Says he is wealthy owning six steamboats, is very strong can walk 60 miles a day. Collects thousands of dollars rent every Saturday night." His condition, complicated by bed sores and a choking episode, began to be closely tracked on May 2, 1874:

> May 2: Growing weaker and duller slowly. Has a fashion of drawing his hands up in his coat sleeves and covering his head with his coat collar, will lie on the bench for hours in this condition, and then get up and walk to the window and look up at the chimney or some other object for a considerable time.
>
> June 10: Became choked upon a large piece of meat became black in the face and was only after some time revived.
>
> June 12: While walking in the hall suddenly fell against the door and has lain in a comatose condition all day.
>
> June 15: Died this morning. Never rallied from his attack. Extensive bed sores found on the 2nd day.[43]

A thousand and three patients died at the asylum during its first two decades. About a third of them were buried in the oldest of the three cemeteries that are tended today on the site.[44] Some families were not interested in retrieving the bodies of their kin from the hospital, and others were undoubtedly simply unable to make the trip necessary—by train or by horse and wagon—to bring the deceased home.

Patients and their families were closely intertwined in the asylum experience. They were deeply connected in regard to the decision to commit a family member, the care patients received at home before commitment, the journey to the asylum, and communications among asylum officers, families, and patients.

A forty-three-year-old single woman with a religious turn of mind stepped off the train in Athens with her brother and a sheriff in February 1874. Depressed and melancholic, she had talked about suicide for the previous six months and "obstinately refused treatment of any kind at home."[45] Her family had tried sending her away to live with her sister for a few weeks, but she remained preoccupied with fears of starvation and of being burned up. She was driven in a hired carriage from the station to the asylum, where she was admitted as Female Patient 49. A few weeks later, a letter arrived from her physician. Writing at the request of her family, the doctor had penned in ink a special note to the asylum superintendent emphasizing his patient's respectable family and her religious piety, noting that she had "many warm friends here who feel a lively interest in her welfare."[46] He had penciled in at the bottom a request for the superintendent to please write with news of his patient.

The bustling Athens train depot was the terminus of the journey of families as they brought their brothers, sisters, children, and parents to the asylum. A collection of establishments—mostly saloons and brothels—lined the dirt street by the station, creating a rough-and-tumble atmosphere into which families exited the train to escort their patients across the river to the institution.[47] Traveling patients judged to be violent were secured by county sheriffs with straitjackets and made the journey with a sheriff's escort. Superintendents of the Athens asylum during the moral treatment years of the nineteenth century were national leaders of the antirestraint movement for patients and insisted on the least restrictive environment possible for their patients; rarely were "sleeves" used at the hospital. County sheriffs, though, used the straitjacket freely in transporting persons to the asylum. Soon-to-be patients traveled weekly on the train to Athens, some arriving in straitjackets or handcuffs.

An elderly widow with failing sight and deficient hearing traveled on the train in a straitjacket, accompanied only by a sheriff. In good health but assessed by family, physician, and judge as violent,

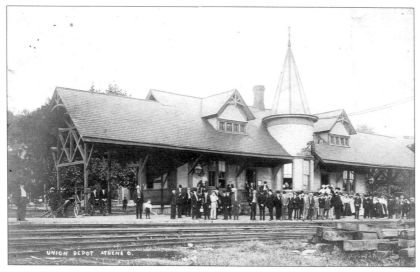

FIGURE 2.6 Union Train Depot in Athens, 1906. *Courtesy of the Athens County Historical Society and Museum.*

destructive, and dangerous, she was sent to the asylum. A fifty-two-year-old unmarried railroad laborer arrived at the Athens train station in handcuffs accompanied by a sheriff. Reluctant to make the journey, he declared to asylum staff when he arrived that he would "get out of here either dead or alive." His asylum physician noted that he was "occasionally abusive and explains his actions by saying that it was not he but some witch speaking through him. . . . [H]e says that his name is Rothschild and that he owns all this building."[48] A woman, native to Germany, arrived in Athens to be hospitalized because of "family trouble."[49] She had traveled on a night train accompanied by a probate judge; both stayed at a hotel in town and reported to the asylum at 9:00 a.m. A forty-eight-year-old woman—fearful of being killed, accusing her family of trying to poison her, and believing in witches—came by train with both her daughter and the local sheriff. A few patients came from Athens, traveling on foot or by wagon. A fifty-six-year-old woman living in the Athens County infirmary was brought by the local sheriff in a horse-drawn wagon. The physician committing her wrote that "she says she has been poisoned a thousand times, believes she is a Queen & c. She is violent at times, the duration of her mental illness of fourteen years. . . . [C]ause is religious excitement."[50]

The dusty rowdiness of the train depot contrasted with the asylum's carefully landscaped grounds, brick towers, elaborate woodwork, and wide carriage drives. Nineteenth-century asylum superintendents sought to create an atmosphere of dignity and safety to reassure the families of patients. The stigma of mental illness and hospitalization sometimes caused families to delay the

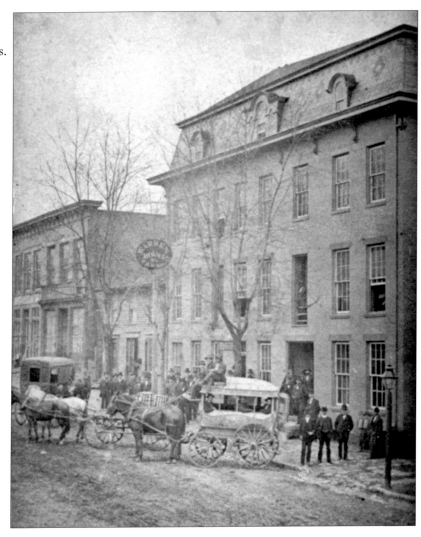

FIGURE 2.7 Warren House, a hotel on Court Street in Athens. Families and others traveling to Athens with persons who had been committed to the asylum might stay overnight in the Warren House or another Athens hotel. *Courtesy of the Mahn Center for Archives and Special Collections, Ohio University Libraries.*

decision to bring a relative to the asylum, thus putting patients at risk. Superintendent William Holden wrote of his worries in his 1879 annual report to the asylum's Board of Trustees:

> I can not too strongly urge upon the friends of the insane the importance of having them admitted to an asylum at their earliest possible opportunity. . . . To some, the idea of consigning a much loved and kind parent, a true and devoted husband or wife, a brother, a sister, or a child to the care of an insane asylum, is repugnant and horrid—a disgrace on the family history. Entertaining this erroneous idea, much valuable time is lost, and the one in whose behalf this sympathy is centered may suffer an irreparable loss. We would have them dispel the idea of an ancient

mad-house, and learn to appreciate the fact that an asylum in this civilized and enlightened age, is a hospital, designed and managed strictly in the interest and for the especial benefit of patients, where they will meet with that close attention, that gentle forbearance, which springs from a proper understanding of their condition.[51]

Families often tried many measures before seeking commitment and making the journey to Athens. They used herbal medicines, tried home remedies, exhausted their own energy, and enlisted the help of other family members. Often they called in physicians who used tonics, bromides, medications to induce sleep, and sedatives. The case of a seventy-three-year-old farmer illustrates the desperation of a family who sought help from several physicians before resorting to home remedies and finally hospitalization. The man was stricken with erysipelas, a bacterial skin infection known also as St. Anthony's fire. Treated today with antibiotics, erysipelas in the nineteenth century frequently led to systemic infection and death. The disease produces a painful swollen rash on the face and legs and may feature hallucinations and seizures. The medical witness filling out the commitment papers for the elderly farmer, Male Patient 200, noted briefly, "Erysipelas . . . the insanity in my opinion has been produced by blood poisoning. After the Physician gave him over to die one of his Sons boiled corn in lye and Applied to him from that point on he Commenced to improve." The man's son had taken up a pencil, related the progress and treatment of his father on a scrap of paper, and conveyed the paper to the asylum superintendent. The fragment was folded in with the official commitment documents, where it has remained for nearly a century and a half. It brings to life the son's struggle before he finally resorted to hospitalization at the asylum.

> Father was insain in the first of his sickness. Father was
> first Doctort by Beers for the liver comanplaint. I think
> the treatment was a calomel with other medicines. Beers
> bing cauld a way and could not attend next we cauld Dr.
> Anderson he doctord him for the liver kitney and dropsy.
> Doctor Leflin said he must dy could not live two weeks,
> Anderson the saim. He stile continued to swell till his hips
> and legs the skin bursted open and his flesh loked nerly a
> churry red and he got entirely helpless. I boled corn in ly
> and let the steem gho to his wounds and the swelling begin

to go Down. I gave him Spice Wood tea to dreank used
embrication oil . . . and held his wounds, and in four weeks
he begin to walk.

Weak, restive, and troubled by hallucinations, however, the farmer
remained ill and on the first day of spring in 1874 was committed to
the asylum, becoming its two hundredth male patient. The family
had to make the 150-mile journey by wagon or rail and must have
done so as a measure of last resort.

The Athens asylum's Superintendent A. B. Richardson was
troubled enough about the care given to mentally ill persons by
their families to recommend to the governor that the state take
charge of all insane persons in Ohio. He had seen too many instances of poor home care provided by friends and families and
cited examples.

> To begin with, every insane person in the State, whether
> in State asylum, private sanitarium, county infirmary or
> private family, should be under efficient State supervision.
> Strange that it should be true, it is nevertheless a fact that
> relatives and friends are not always safe custodians of the
> insane. Within the past few days one instance has come
> under my notice where a daughter had been confined
> for twelve years or more, by a mother, in a basement
> room necessarily with defective light and ventilation,
> and another mother writes us, after we had received her
> daughter, that she had found it necessary at home to put
> a strap about her daughter's waist to which she confined
> her hands, and had also found it a necessity, on some
> occasions, to tie her feet together.[52]

Superintendents complained, however, that too many families
brought their elderly members to the asylum when they should be
cared for at home. Dr. Rutter noted, for example,

> The admissions show a very large number of very aged
> persons. Old men and women who have been bruised
> and battered by toil and anxiety, and who finally succumb
> to the combined attacks of old age and hard work. First
> sleepless, then peevish, irritable and peculiar, they soon
> become a source of annoyance to their friends, and are
> adjudged insane, and hustled off to the asylum. Surely
> many a pathetic story could be woven from the meshes
> furnished by these examples of sorrow and suffering. They

tell the sad story of usefulness outlived, and too often of filial ingratitude. Many of them, after having toiled and struggled, and denied themselves the comforts and often the necessaries of life, in order to provide against the time when old age would render them helpless, and also to provide a "start" in the world for their children, become a household burden, and the childishness and querulousness of old age is made the pretext for removing them to the Asylum. Here, among strangers . . . they droop and die.[53]

In the 1880s, generally only about three in twenty of the asylum's patients were age sixty and over. But superintendents were likely discouraged by their inability to cure the dementia or poor health with which the elderly patients arrived, having been committed by their children or grandchildren. The commitment documents of elderly patients reveal the condition in which they were brought by their families. Five family members testified to a probate judge in Marietta, Ohio, of the insanity of a fifty-nine-year-old woman. Living alone and infirm, she was committed with this description from the family physician: "Mrs. _____ is quiet, lives alone, doing her own work, though quite infirm. Talks coherently, but sometimes refers to visual hallucinations or certain insane delusions as to her bodily ailments that become matters of belief and indicate a disordered mind." She entered the asylum as Female Patient 345 a few days later. A sixty-five-year-old man, Male Patient 31, was committed by his children after ten years of poor health and a recent attack of neuralgia (nerve pain). A seventy-one-year-old widow of "limited education" described as a mother of four children and a homemaker of "amiable disposition," had suffered from "senile dementia" for two years. Her friends having abandoned her, her son cared for her in his home for fifteen months before committing her. The medical witness found her depressed, unable to sleep but with a "pleasant natural disposition."[54]

In fact, nineteenth-century state asylum superintendents had little control over the kinds of patients families sought to have admitted to their institutions, and few were turned away.[55] County judges and local physicians determined whether a person was insane, so community norms and judgments determined what persons were sent to the asylum for admission. Concerned about maintaining public safety and relieving burdens of care of their constituents, county probate judges convened inquests into insanity in their chambers in the county seat and made determinations about insanity in regard to its impact on physical, social, and economic life.[56] In general, violent behavior, destruction of property, and low economic productivity of mentally ill persons increased the likelihood of their hospitalization.

Patients with seizure disorders, known in the nineteenth century simply as epilepsy, were regarded by asylum physicians as a special challenge. In 1874, a twenty-seven-year-old woman was committed because of seizures, which a local physician serving as medical witness had determined was not epilepsy. Ohio's commitment documents required a physician to certify whether or not a prospective patient had epilepsy; a determination of epilepsy was much less likely to result in hospitalization. Asylum physicians had little idea of how to treat seizure disorders, and the seemingly random disturbance of seizures was upsetting to asylum routine, patients, and staff. This young woman's affliction was judged to have been caused by falling off her horse into an icy creek while menstruating. She had been hospitalized in the asylum at Dayton, Ohio, for a few years and then sent home.[57] The young woman, hospitalized again, was accompanied by her mother on her journey to the asylum, and her commitment papers included a letter from the county probate judge with a personal request to help out the parents by accepting the daughter as a patient. The judge wrote to Superintendent Gundry, "Dear Sir: Enclosed I send you papers in case of _____[,] one of your old Dayton patients—who has been in bad condition for some time. I hope you will be able to take her back as she is a great charge at home with her aged parents."[58]

Inability to contribute to the welfare and well-being of family and community contributed to a family's decision to commit one of its members. Women were committed when their illness prevented them from taking care of their families. A forty-seven-year-old woman from the Ohio River town of Marietta had taken to her bed for nine months, refusing to see anyone. The medical witness to her insanity wrote, "Does not want to see anyone, inclines to discard most all of her own relations. Lays abed most of the time with head covered up, especially so if any one comes in where she is. Duration eight years at that time had an attack which lasted several months then got better and went on well until eight or nine months ago when she had another attack which continues to the present." She was hospitalized by her family in the asylum at Athens a few months after it opened.[59] A twenty-six-year-old mother, incapacitated by anxiety about caring for her five children, whom she had borne in the space of six years, was hospitalized by her husband. The physician who assisted the husband in committing her determined, "The present exciting cause (of her insanity) is over anxiety about her children."[60]

Some families brought more than one of their own to the asylum. In the instance of a sixty-year-old lawyer (Male Patient 706) from the Ohio River town of Portsmouth, the commitment of his son (Male Patient 701) worsened the condition of this elderly father so that both were admitted to the asylum within a month of each other. The son soon recovered and went home, but the father remained at the asylum, dying there in 1887.[61] He left a collection of vivid and forceful letters written to his family at home, which were retained and filed by asylum staff.[62] In one he described a journey to the asylum, which seems to be a reflection on his own experience blended with that of his son. It conveys his feelings of despair about both.

> I on this beautiful Lords day Summer morning. (The third Sunday in Trinity). Informing you of my continued good health and mental intellectual enjoyment. I have made another retrograde movement. I now occupy a single room. Without any one to interfere with my meditations. Which is congenial to my wishes. I am however in what they call Ward Fifteen "Athens Ohio". . . . George took [my son] by those two other "insane Men" from Portsmouth. He knew nothing of them: Of the ass . . . that Jesus Christ: Rode into Jerusalem . . . Aaron before Robert . . . judge of the "Court of Reprobates"! When and where he perjured himself . . . and the devil knows how many more. I left the sheriff's office on the morning of the eighth of August at nine minutes or near that in company of Sheriff Rheinegar and Barny Aaron Moses! (a railroad conductor) and went to the depot . . . and took the ten o'clock train for Albany: at Webster: or Concord! Barney Aaron Groseby! Came about from the "car of juggernaut" and conducted the Pullman Car . . . to Athens & via of Hamden, Marshfield, Athens. Bringing . . . at Albany Ohio and New York. He stayed all night in Albany Ohio. The next day the ninth he passed through Ward eighteen at about ten o'clock. And I have never heard from him since only by your mother. Last May a year agone: A Guilty conscience . . . no accused. . . . And what has since transpired. Forgive and forget it is better. To fling every feeling aside. Than allow the deep cankering fester of revenge in they breast to abide. . . .

Render therefore unto Casear! The things that are Caesars: And to God the things that are God's.[63]

His long and elaborate letters home reflected on family, politics, and religion and included references to classical scholarship. In a letter written in late August 1880, he asked his son to take him home: "Why do you not come after me? Get a writ of habeas corpus a search warrant of reprieve and attachment. Bring Sheriff or take me from my Gaolers . . . but I have lived and have not lived in vain. My mind has never lost its force. My blood is fine. . . . Write me a letter."[64] Later he rebuked his family for failing to inform him of the death of a niece:

> Is it True? Did Sara die? And go to her Father god? Oh! How cruelly wicked you all have been. In keeping me in ignorance. Of her death, for I have said many hard things. That I would not have said. Had I knew she was Dead. . . . Remember. That "Blessed are the dead, that die in the Lord. That from henceforth! Yea sayeth the Spirit they rest from their labors. And their words to follow them. There is no death: the stars go down. To rise on some . . . shore: And bright the heaven's jeweld crown O they shine forevermore." . . . And that Sara died last spring! Why had I never been apprised of the death. Is shrouded in impenetrable Mystery![65]

He continued to reproach his family and ask them to take him home, sometimes ruminating about politics.

> [My son] was coming after me, and soon as he got his corn planted. He has been coming ever since! And has not got there yet. He was here, four or five years ago. And moved off and left me here. Where I do nothing whatever mentally or physically. And every man on earth or heaven knows it that has a thimble full of brains. . . . The Presidential Election of November, 1876! Between Butler, Tilden and Hayes.[66] You must remember the Louisiana and Florida Returning Boards. The Black boards. And Bulletin Boards. The Electoral Colleges. And the States that voted by their Deputies. Delegates Legislatures. General Assemblies. The seventh of August I last saw you. Do you know where San Louis Potosi San Christobell Spain is? What Latitude or Longitude? How long since you was at Rock Island Illinois? Or Sidney

and Mellbourne Australia? Pall Mall England? Did you remember The Wheel = right to you Aaron [Burr?]. . . . I make this proposition to you jointly and severally: come and see me and I will accompany you Home, paying all traveling expenses, each way. Your Father.[67]

The decision of a family to commit one of its members to the asylum at Athens depended on several factors, and the asylum was generally not the first choice of treatment. A family's choice to seek a declaration of insanity from the county probate judge, which required appearing in the judge's chambers with a medical witness, was often delayed because of the stigma of mental illness and the length of the journey required to reach Athens.[68] Families tried other measures, including treatment by local physicians, help from extended family, use of home remedies, and sometimes willingness to try desperate measures. While the work required to supervise and care for a family member with a chronic mental illness could be long and wearing, most families were willing to try for a while. They were much less likely to delay with physically unmanageable family members. Husbands, wives, mothers, fathers, and children who were deemed dangerous to family, community, and themselves—threatening and attempting murder and suicide—were not tolerated for long by families and communities. Families were also more likely to seek commitment for one of their relatives when the mentally ill person was no longer able to help support the welfare of the family. Women who could no longer care for their children or the household—lying abed or paralyzed by anxiety over the welfare of her children—were brought to the asylum by husbands or sisters. Men who had become unable to contribute to the family—depressed, morose, and unable to help with family—were brought by friends and wives to the asylum.

Commitment decisions were made locally, in the county seats of the twenty-eight-county area served by the Athens asylum. Probate judges and sheriffs concerned about supporting their constituencies and maintaining order and safety in their communities heard the requests brought by families and their physicians and made legal determinations of insanity. For the most part, anyone brought to the asylum would be admitted as a patient.

Once patients were committed, however, the asylum's superintendents played a significant role with their families. Superintendents sent letters home briefing families on the condition of their patient and their prospects for recovery. Although some families took patients home before they were determined to be well, others came and got them only after the asylum notified them that their patients were recovered. Superintendents sent letters to families asking them to provide clothing for their patients, detailing in their letters the types of clothing needed. When patients wrote letters home, asylum staff read them and made decisions not to mail at least some of them and instead retained them in the superintendents' files of correspondence. Families wrote asking for news of their family members, inquiring whether they might visit them in the asylum, and sending bad news to be conveyed by a physician. Superintendents responded to the letters and made decisions about whether and how to convey these family messages.

During the asylum's moral treatment years (1874–93), 3,556 patients were discharged; a quarter of them were readmitted. Male Patient 9, a forty-nine-year-old farmer committed by his wife, was admitted and discharged twice within the space of fourteen months. The casebook follows his progress:

> Patient history [January 1874]: The exciting event was the sale of a farm and the duration of his symptoms eighteen months. He has been despondent and could not sleep. Thinks his family will come to want. Tried to hang himself. Has habit of pulling out his hair so that he is almost bald in some areas of the head.
>
> February 1874: Gradually improving.
>
> May 1874: Very much improved. Works outside and is about well enough to go home.
>
> June 14, 1874: Taken home well.
>
> June 25, 1874: Returned by wife who stated that after he got home all energy left him and he would lie in bed all day hardly getting up to eat one meal a day. And would say that he could not make a living and that they would all starve.
>
> July 30, 1874: As well as when taken home.
>
> February 18, 1875: Was discharged this morning. Wife came to see him last evening and they slipped off to bed together in the fireman's room.[69]

We are left to guess whether the patient had recovered or was judged well enough to go home because he had slipped off with his wife.

THREE

ARCHITECTURE

"Space, Light and Air to Each Patient"

The brick masons paused in their work. It was time to change positions on the muddy site, where walls three bricks thick were rising off their stone foundations, nearly reaching the height of the bottom of the first-floor windows. It was April 1868, and the stone- and brickwork of the cellars and basement was complete and ready to support the massive brick exterior wall, trimmed with Buena Vista freestone that had been quarried in southern Ohio.[1] The building measured 853 feet long in a direct line, the recesses and projections of its footprint a little over three-quarters of a mile.[2] A large building in any location, for rural Athens the new asylum was massive, far greater in size and scope than any building for a hundred miles or more in any direction. Its sturdy load-bearing masonry construction, typical of the nineteenth century, featured stone and brick walls two and three feet thick at their base.

Brick masons rotated their positions on this type of building frequently so that the small idiosyncrasies and techniques making up the look or "signature" of each man would blend into a coherent whole. The men on the job site for the new asylum had been laying bricks as fast as they were being made, but with that spring's snow, followed by rain, the brick-making operation had been seriously delayed. The manufacturers, D. W. H. Day and James W. Sands, were having a hard time making good on their commitment to the trustees to deliver eighteen and a half million bricks. The bricks were being manufactured on the construction site on top of the ridge above the Hocking River using southeastern Ohio shale and clay dug straight from the site. Ten years later, the clay in this region would support a thriving brick paver industry. But in contrast to paver bricks, which were extruded from presses and baked, these construction bricks for

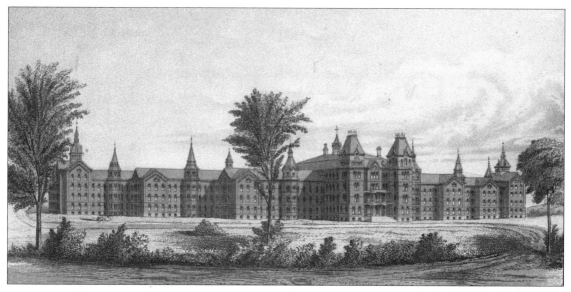

FIGURE 3.1
Lithograph of a drawing of the front elevation of the plan for the asylum prepared by Cleveland architect Levi Scofield. The central administrative core was flanked by the male *(left)* and female *(right)* patient wings. *Board of Trustees of the Southeastern Lunatic Asylum, 1872 annual report, 1.*

the asylum were still being made by the old method: formed outdoors in wooden molds and fired in beehive kilns fueled with coal.[3]

Hundreds of expert carpenters, masons, plasterers, mosaic tile setters, laborers, and other craftsmen worked for six years to build the Athens Lunatic Asylum and finish its interior spaces, its High Victorian Italianate style featuring windowed towers. From a construction point of view, its vernacular craftsmanship is brilliant.[4] Fifty stonecutters and masons and seventy-five quarriers and laborers were hired by contractor William McAboy to excavate the cellars and do all the stonework.[5] Contractors in Cincinnati provided slate roofing, cut and hauled marble, built iron gutters and ornamental cornices, and contracted for yellow pine flooring as well as joist and roof timbers.[6] Cincinnati industrialist Miles Greenwood, who made wrought ironwork for buildings as well as wrought-iron and cast-iron hardware, fulfilled the needs for iron-

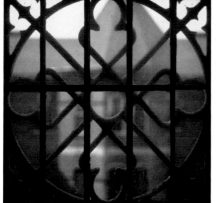

work. The floor joists of heavy timber were set in place by Henry O'Bleness and his partner, W. W. McCoy. The interior spaces were painted with a glowing palette of colors such as vermillion (a deep red-orange), burnt umber, chrome green, chrome yellow, Prussian blue, raw umber, rose pink, yellow

FIGURE 3.2 The iron security grilles in front of the windows were disguised by the architect as decorative mandalas. Each floor of the asylum had its own slightly different grille design. Shown is the design for the third floor. *Photograph courtesy of George Eberts.*

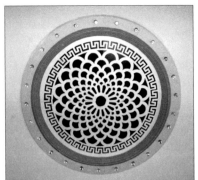

FIGURE 3.3 (*left*) Ceiling ornament from the free-standing amusement hall, built in 1900. *Photograph courtesy of Doug McCabe.*

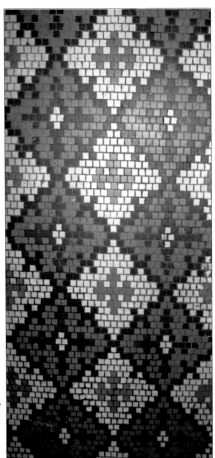

FIGURE 3.4 (*right*) Original tile floor in the center administrative section of the building. *Photograph courtesy of Doug McCabe.*

FIGURE 3.5 (*below*) Stencil detail for the ceiling of the original amusement hall, now referred to as the ballroom, located within the central administrative core of the original building. *Photograph courtesy of Doug McCabe.*

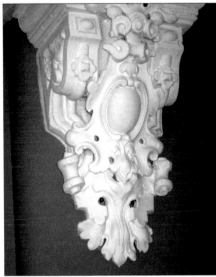

FIGURE 3.6 (*above*) Interior architectural detail in administrative section, now renovated space for the Kennedy Museum of Art of Ohio University. *Photograph courtesy of Doug McCabe.*

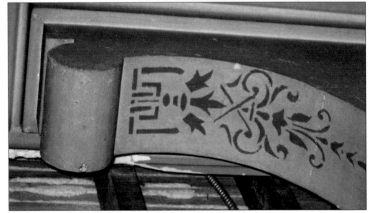

ochre, Persian brown, and Tuscan red. Mr. D. W. H. Day worked to fulfill his sixty-thousand-dollar brick-making contract. And O'Bleness completed the building's carpentry and other woodwork, towers, and connecting buildings.

O'Bleness walked across the huge job site, observing the brick masons shift their positions. Having taken full charge of the carpentry from his former partner, he meant to get on with the interior work so that he would be in a position to bid on the contract for the ornate ventilation towers high atop the building. At present, he was assembling and organizing his crew for finishing the basement, which was now under cover. At twenty-seven, Henry was a man with complete confidence in his ability to take on this contract. Born in the Ohio River town of Belpre, he lived with his parents until he was nineteen, learning his father's trade, that of a carpenter and joiner. He came from a line of American builders who had lived in the New York City area since before the Revolutionary War. During the Civil War, O'Bleness served as a sergeant in the 148th Ohio National Guard, and he also worked in the construction and lumber industry along the Ohio River.

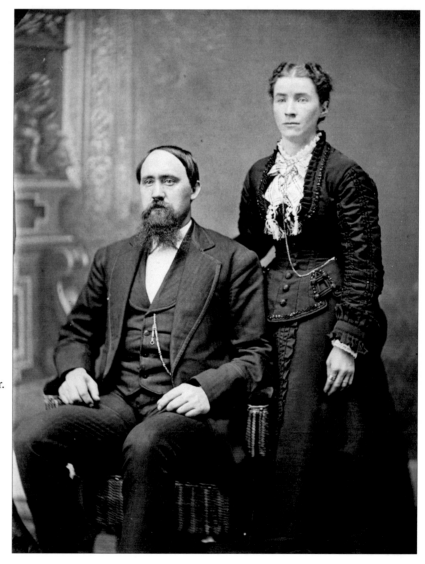

FIGURE 3.7 Builder Henry O'Bleness and his wife, Josephine. Mr. O'Bleness completed the woodwork for the construction of the asylum as well as its ventilation towers. *Courtesy of the Mahn Center for Archives and Special Collections, Ohio University Libraries.*

Obtaining the woodwork and carpentry contract from the asylum trustees was his first big project, and he would make the most of it.

Henry O'Bleness's success at completing the woodwork for the trustees of the asylum allowed him to settle permanently in Athens and become the town's major builder. Within fifteen years, he had built the town hall, the Athens County Courthouse, numerous office and market buildings, buildings at Ohio University, and private homes. The asylum's trustees later awarded him contracts for its additions: an icehouse, a new storehouse, and new patient dining rooms. When he received the contract for constructing the asylum's towers in 1871, he married Miss Josephine Shearer from Belpre, and they went on to have four children together. A Master Mason, he was also an astute businessman; his construction firm laid the foundation for family wealth, which became in the twentieth century a source of community philanthropy in Athens.[7]

Henry O'Bleness and his fellow contractors and builders were creating what would become a visual record of more than a century of psychiatry. The distinctive feature of the original building's footprint is the stepped-back wings, designed to capture light and fresh air. This plan, conceived by Dr. Thomas Story Kirkbride for the Pennsylvania Hospital for the Insane, also served to segregate patients by gender and by "class." At the ends of the two main wings were the back wards, which in the nineteenth century housed patients of the class described in the psychiatric language of the times as noisy, destructive, excited, demented, or violent.[8] Asylum

FIGURE 3.8 Plan of the Athens Lunatic Asylum prepared by architect Levi Scofield. The winglike extensions from the central administrative core are features of the Kirkbride plan. Patients considered quiet and well-behaved were housed closest to the central administrative core; the most physically or verbally expressive patients were in the far wings. *Board of Trustees of the Southeastern Lunatic Asylum of Ohio, 1872 annual report, 2.*

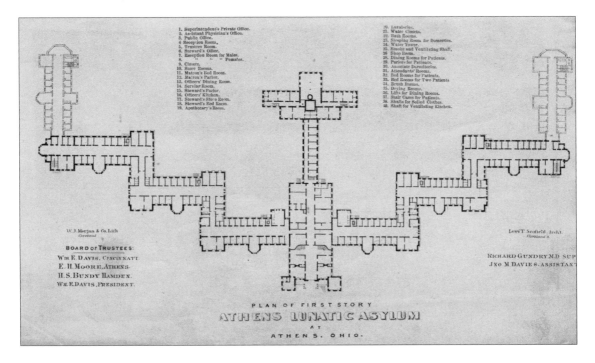

physicians believed that the presence of more agitated patients had a negative effect on quieter patients, so they were isolated in the far ends of the building. This arrangement also kept the sounds and sights of the excited patients far from the living quarters of the staff in the central part of the building. For in a Kirkbride asylum, most of the staff lived as well as worked in the building.

Four years later, Dr. Richard Gundry, superintendent of the state's Southern Asylum at Dayton and friend of Governor Rutherford B. Hayes, stood with his back to the river and studied the asylum. It was a cold November day in 1872, and although lawn grass had been sowed and evergreen seedlings ordered, the site was bare. Flakes of snow blew in his face; up on the hill to his right, a few yellow and orange-pink leaves clung to the sycamore and sassafras trees. The brickwork for the central administration building and the extension wings was finally complete, all the interiors were plastered, most of the plumbing was completed, the roofing was finished, and the boilers for the steam heat would soon be in place. Inside, the flooring was being laid. O'Bleness had finished several of the ventilating towers, the cisterns were ready, the gas pipes were laid, and most of the stone flooring was laid in the kitchen, laundry, and basement. The year before, Dr. Gundry had chosen pictures for the walls of the wards of the asylum; this year, he had purchased reference books for the library of the physicians who would work there. He had been retained by the trustees to review the progress of construction and make recommendations for completion. In this he was assisted by Mr. John M. Davies of Athens, who had been in charge of construction since the cornerstone laying in 1868. Gundry's conclusions, written to the trustees, echo Sir Henry Wotton's principles of well-building known to any architect today: "commodity, firmness and delight."[9] That is, he believed the building suited its purpose, would withstand wear and tear, and was visually pleasing:

> Such are the principal features of the building, now
> approaching completion, to which your anxious and
> assiduous efforts have been so freely given. . . . [T]he exterior
> of the building is certainly pleasing to the eye, and conforms
> to the benevolent purpose to which it is devoted. No gloomy
> aspect will terrify the patient as he approaches and enters
> this building, and whoever considers the importance of
> the first impressions made upon a bewildered and fearful

sufferer, as he enters what will prove him a prison or a home, will not think these are slight matters. Your architect, Mr. Scofield, deserves the highest credits for the results of his professional skill in planning and arranging this great structure, so as to combine the essential features of an hospital with the strength required for the peculiar class of invalids to be treated, without throwing over them the gloomy and forbidding aspects of a prison. What he so ably and tastefully designed has generally been admirably carried out by the contractors who have done the work.[10]

Dr. Gundry, though, was concerned about four things: fire, water, furnishings, and a restraint-free environment for patients.[11] Topmost in his mind was a terrible fire four years previous at the Central Ohio Lunatic Asylum in Columbus, which had destroyed the building and killed six patients.[12] He recommended fireproofing the attic, where most large institutional fires started and were quickly spread when flaming attic floors fell. The floors and ceiling joists of the new asylum consisted only of pine boards; Gundry recommended building another floor over the attic floor of iron arches and joists covered with concrete to contain any fire starting in that area.

Water was his next concern. The trustees had planned for springs on the grounds to provide all the water for the asylum. Gundry judged them inadequate because of their scattered location and their drought-depleted state. Noting that the asylum would need more than thirty thousand gallons per day, he recommended building a reservoir on a hill of the grounds, to be filled by the river below. A well at the bottom of the hill would filter the water, and it would be pumped to the reservoir by means of a steam pump. The water would enter the building by way of pipes laid around the building and would be sufficient in the case of fire emergency.

As to providing for the interior of the building, Dr. Gundry recommended placing orders for the furniture and other items as soon as possible, because they would need to be made to order.

Finally, the superintendent was committed to creating an environment as free as possible of patient restraints. He felt that building strong rooms would do nothing but encourage their use. He therefore recommended not completing the plans for a return wing in each of the third sections of each side of the building fitted out with "strong rooms for excited patients."[13] He suggested instead adding a small section of wards on each side especially designed for excited patients. Gundry specified that these should be for a small number of patients and made as appealing as possible, with special additions for physically violent patients, such as windows with shutters sliding into the walls and a veranda at the end of the corridor for fresh air for those who were not allowed to walk outside. An alternative would be adapting some of the existing rooms in this manner.

The board of trustees recommended to the governor that the state provide funds right away for the fireproofing and provision for water. Without the recommended reservoir and pumps to access water from the Hocking River, there would be just a trickle of water for the asylum, and the recent fire at the Columbus asylum was fresh in the minds and imaginations of all. The springs later became an ornamental feature of the landscape rather than a source of drinking water. The small wards designed and built specially to humanely provide for excited patients the trustees put on hold. With an estimated cost of $100,000, the construction of these wards was left to the new, managing board of trustees that would come into service in two years. The initial trustees hoped to open the institution to patients in seven months, July 1873, and turn the management of the asylum over to the new board then.

Dr. Gundry started for the hill with the sycamore and sassafras trees. He wished to pace out the distance from its top to the asylum in order to make a closer estimate of the cost of running a water pipe from the proposed reservoir. Tomorrow he would meet with architect Levi Scofield, who was on his way to Athens from Cleveland. Together they would meet with the trustees to discuss the water and fireproofing engineering considerations.

FIGURE 3.9 View of the asylum in 1875 from the village of Athens *(left background)*. Villagers watched from town as the building took form on the hill across the river. Tours were conducted for the public the month before it opened. Originally published in Lake, *Atlas of Athens County, Ohio. Courtesy of the Mahn Center for Archives and Special Collections, Ohio University Libraries.*

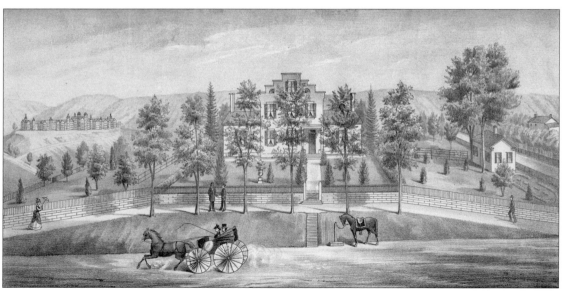

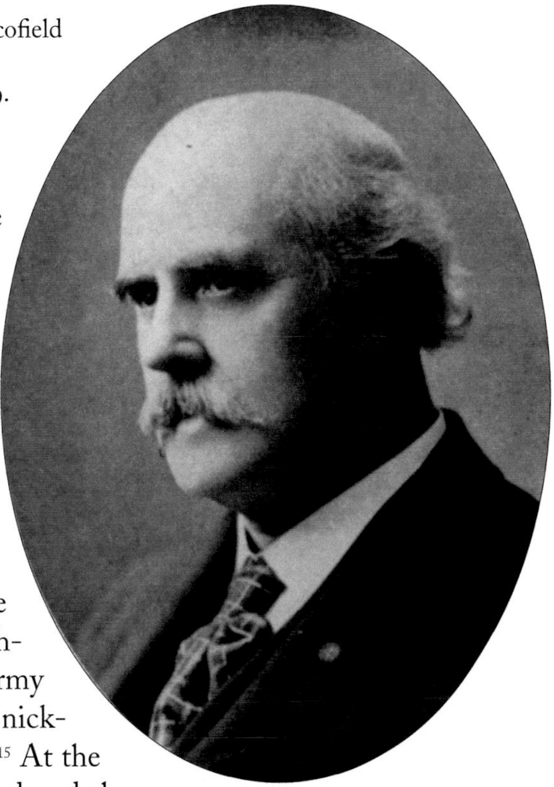

FIGURE 3.10 Cleveland architect Levi Tucker Scofield designed the Athens Lunatic Asylum. Originally published in *Progressive Men of Northern Ohio*, 219. *Courtesy of the Mahn Center for Archives and Special Collections, Ohio University Libraries.*

Captain Levi Tucker Scofield, the youngest of three generations of Cleveland builders and architects, had enlisted in the army at the outbreak of the Civil War and served in the 103rd Ohio Volunteer Infantry. Among the Union troops who pursued Morgan and his Raiders through Ohio and West Virginia, Scofield was appointed aide-de-camp and engineer on the staff of General J. D. Cox and participated in Chickamauga, the siege upon Atlanta, the defeat of Hood at Nashville, and the capture of Raleigh.[14] His army engineering skills had gained him the nickname among the troops of "Old Topog."[15] At the war's end, he returned home to Cleveland and then moved to New York City for a short time, working as an architectural draftsman and cultivating his skills as a sculptor. The year 1867 was an important one for the young architect: at the age of twenty-five he married Elizabeth Clark Wright and received the commission for the Athens Lunatic Asylum, his first major project. On the strength of his work in Athens, Scofield built a national reputation for designing Victorian institutions such as the National Soldiers and Sailors Orphanage in Xenia, Ohio; the North Carolina Penitentiary at Raleigh; and the new Asylum for the Insane in Columbus. His family and business connections gained him access to wealthy Cleveland industrialists, such as John D. Rockefeller, who became one of Scofield's golfing partners.

The Kirkbride Plan

For the asylum at Athens, Scofield had prepared drawings of the plan and elevation of the building as well as all the specifications and documentation for the materials and construction of the building. He made trips in 1867 and 1868 to Athens from Cleveland, a journey of several days. Before assigning the contract, the asylum trustees had determined that the asylum should be built in accordance with the Kirkbride plan, late nineteenth-century psychiatry's "gold standard" of treatment. The trustees had investigated public buildings and charitable institutions known to be the best of their time, studying particularly their methods of heating and ventilation.[16] They had given the commission to Mr. Scofield with detailed instructions and examples from Kirkbride asylums in other locations. Dr. Richardson was pleased with the result; indeed, he had to agree with the assessment of the trustees that the building was "second to none in this country in its appointments, conveniences, healthfulness and beauty of location."[17] Dr. Gundry described in detail the design of the asylum and the functions of its spaces, beginning with its central administrative core.

> The Administration Building is four stories in height, and comprises a front and rear division. The first includes, on the first floor, an entrance hall sixteen feet wide and fifty-five long, on each side of which are the offices of superintendent, assistant physicians and steward, and general reception room for visitors, and the large stairways to the stories above. The second story of this division contains the compartments of the medical superintendent. The third and fourth stories comprise similar rooms for the other officers of the institution. In the rear division of the administration building, a central hall twelve feet wide, leads from the front to the rear, on either side of which are the passages to the patients' wards. In the basement of this division are placed the kitchens, sculleries, and other domestic rooms for the general household, and beneath these are cellars. On the first floor are the dining-rooms and kitchen of the officers, reception rooms for friends of patients, and general store-room. On the second floor the central hall leads to the amusement hall, 66 feet by 42 feet, and twenty-eight feet in height, occupying both second and third stories. Above this room, in the fourth story, is a room of similar size, sixteen feet high, designed for religious services. Besides these rooms, there are on each of these stories two rooms for reading, sewing and other purposes, and on every floor bath-rooms. A stairway leads from the basement to the second story in this division.[18]

The central administrative building separating the male and female wings reflected the authoritarian nature and structure of

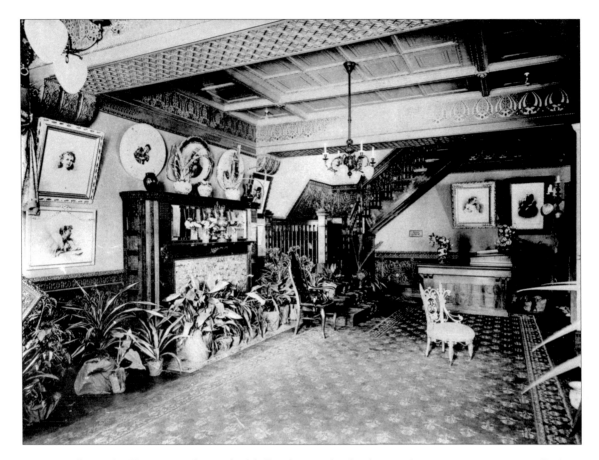

FIGURE 3.11 Parlor in the administrative section of the building. *Courtesy of the Mahn Center for Archives and Special Collections, Ohio University Libraries.*

a well-to-do Victorian household. It also embodied moral treatment's hopes for the curative function of a regular, harmonious environment with a regimen that would influence patients to internalize the behaviors of a well-ordered household. With private offices and public parlors on the ground floor, the upper floors of the administrative core contained living and dining spaces for the officers, a chapel, and the large amusement hall. Here the superintendent, assistant physicians, and steward lived with their families, dined, conducted business, and met with the families of patients. Here also were conducted cultural entertainments and weekly church services led by local ministers and priests.

The superintendent lived with his family in a spacious high-ceilinged second-floor apartment overlooking the institution's front entrance; his office was downstairs adjoining the wide tile entrance hall. His location was emblematic of his role and status as a "stern, authoritarian, yet loving and concerned father . . . [while] the ideal hospital itself was seen as a cohesive and closely knit family, within whose confines the superintendent would treat patients with consideration and respect in the hope of eliciting a response in kind."[19] Behind and beneath this administrative core were work and living spaces for "domestics"—attendants, cooks, laundresses, and bakers—as well as the heating and mechanical systems supporting the building. The original plan had located the huge heating boilers in the rear of the administration building, next to employee quarters, but for safety reasons Dr. Gundry had recommended their placement farther to the rear.

> Under the wings is a basement connecting with the kitchens and basement of the administration building, in which will be the railroad for the conveyance of food to the dumb-waiters of the dining-rooms in each ward, and the chambers for the steam coils and pipes connecting them to heat the wards above. In the rear of the administration building is a series of buildings, comprising connecting building, laundry building and boiler-house. The connecting building contains a long corridor continuous with the central hall of administration building, having on one side eight rooms for domestics or other purposes. In the basement is a similar corridor, and also passage for steam pipes, &c. Below this is the air duct for supplying air to steam coils of main building. The laundry building has two stories and a basement. In the basement will be the washing, drying and ironing rooms, also the engine-rooms and bakery. The back part of this basement was intended for the boilers, but these now occupy a separate building. In the first and second stories, over this, are rooms designed for workshops. The remainder of these stories will be devoted to rooms for domestics. In the centre of this building is situated the water tower, 68 feet high, containing four large iron tanks capable of holding 8,000 gallons of water. These are supported upon iron beams. Still further in the rear is the boiler house, built especially for the six boilers for heating the building. The reasons for removing them from the quarters designed for them are obvious. In case of explosion, or other accident, the lives of so many would be exposed to so much risk which it is not right to induce them to incur. Moreover, the comfort of the employes would be sadly interfered with from the great heat of the boilers, immediately beneath them, in the same building.[20]

Over the next few years, improvements were made to the domestic spaces. For instance, the storeroom, located under the

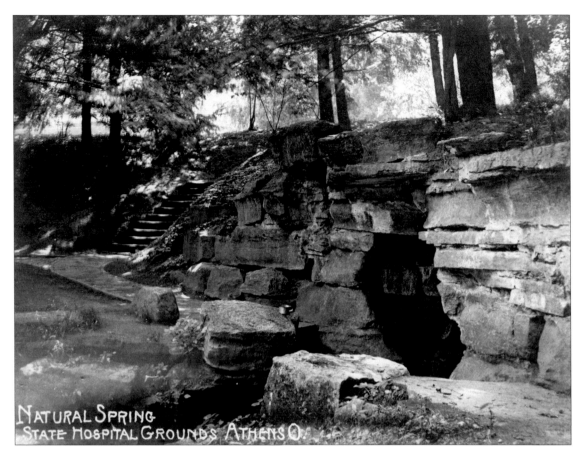

NATURAL SPRING
STATE HOSPITAL GROUNDS ATHENS O.

corridor connecting the main building with the kitchen, employee dining rooms and quarters, was continually damp and too small—"in every way unfit for the purpose."[21] To make matters worse, the heated air from the furnaces was vitiated by the odors of vegetables, meats, and fish over which it passed on its way to the main building; moreover, the boxed-in heating tubes provided a haven for rats. A veranda, urgently needed to protect the front of the building from the wear and tear of weather and requested of the governor continually for ten years, was built in 1893, thus, with the fountain, completing the front façade as it is today.

Fanning out from the central administration building were the two wings housing patients. These spaces, three and four stories in height, contained wards of individual rooms and dormitories for patients all situated along fifteen-foot-wide hallways. Each ward featured a large parlor with a tall bay window through which morning light streamed, a small dining room, bathrooms, lavatory, and water closets. An essential part of moral treatment philosophy, and one manifested in bricks and mortar, was the ward system. Nineteenth-century asylum psychiatry classified patients and segregated them geographically within the asylum; patients who were

FIGURE 3.12 The postcard shows a view of a spring with stone steps and a wall constructed by asylum employees and patients in the nineteenth century. Remnants are visible today. *Courtesy of the Mahn Center for Archives and Special Collections, Ohio University Libraries.*

less actively disturbed were housed together, for example, apart from the troublesome influence of those patients who were more violent or noisy. The goal of classification was to provide an environment in which the patient might be influenced positively by those around him or her.[22] The building's architecture was an important tool for managing patient behavior. For if a patient failed to conform to the expectations for behavior and conduct in his or her ward, s/he might be moved to a ward where such behavior was tolerated but social amenities were restricted.[23]

> On either side of the administration building in the wings are the wards for patients. Each wing is of three stories in height, except at the end, where a fourth story is placed over part of the third section. Each wing is divided into three sections, connected together, but receding in echelon. Thus ten wards are made on each side, providing for the classification to that extent of each sex. Each ward contains a central corridor, fifteen feet wide, with the rooms opening into it on each side. In the center of the front part of each ward is the parlor, a handsome room, 24 by 16 feet, with bay window. A dining-room and associate dormitories, and bath-rooms, lavatory and water-closets are attached to every ward. An iron stairway leads in every section from basement to attic, and communicates with each floor therein. Thus it will be seen that on every floor there are six wards for patients. The single bed-rooms are about 9 feet by 11 feet, and vary in height from twelve to fifteen feet. The associate dormitories vary in size from ten feet by twenty feet, to twenty by twenty feet. Reckoning each single bed-room to be occupied by one patient, and the dormitories by the numbers they are designed to accommodate without improper crowding, there will be in these wards ample room for 572 patients, as follows: in 282 single rooms, 282 persons; in 61 associated dormitories, 290 persons.[24]

Thomas Kirkbride in his treatise on the architecture of moral treatment specified forced ventilation—fresh air passing over steam-heated pipes or plates—to provide the most healthful indoor atmosphere possible. Kirkbride, in describing the architectural and design aspects of moral treatment, took pains to describe a proper boiler operation placed, for safety, at a distance of at least one hundred feet from the main building.[25] Dr. Gundry in his inspection and description of the new building detailed its heating and ventilation.

> The whole building will be heated by steam, generated by six boilers, and conveyed to steam coils enclosed in chambers immediately attached to the flue of the room intended to be heated. Under the wards these chambers are placed in the rooms and communicate with the external air, and there is a distinct chamber to each flue. In the wards, the dining-rooms, parlors and attendants rooms will also be supplied with direct radiation, so that both direct and indirect radiation will be relied upon. In the main building, the chambers containing the steam coils derive their air from an air shaft into which pure air will pass from without. This part of the building is also largely supplied with fire-places in the various rooms, the oldest and best mode of heating and ventilation yet discovered. In the rooms for domestics direct radiation will be used. Wherever the room is to be warmed by indirect radiation, the heated air is brought in near the ceiling and the ventilating flues, open near the floor and also near the ceilings, except where they would be too close to the hot air openings. In this way, it is believed, that the atmosphere will be made more equable and less interrupted by the opening and shutting of doors and windows, while the annoyance of stuffing the hot air flues with torn papers and shreds, so constantly observed in the wards of the insane, is entirely obviated. The ventilating flues, passing from the upper and lower portions of the rooms to the attics, open into the corridors there, whence the foul air is drawn to the ventilating towers in the centre of each section. These towers will contain direct radiators for this purpose. All the water closets are ventilated downwards by air ducts communicating directly from the soil pipe to the smoke stack.[26]

The asylum at Athens employed an engineer, firemen, and coal-wheelers to run this heating system. The skills and watchfulness of the engineer in monitoring fuel, temperature, and pressure of the boilers were critical for the safety of the asylum community all living together in the complex. These men also tended two huge fans located in the basement. Made in Pittsburgh of gleaming brass, the fans circulated air up the shafts that ran throughout the asylum, and most especially to all patient rooms, to create the ventilation so important to the architecture of moral treatment.

Richard Gundry started back down the hill he had just climbed, pacing off the distance from its top to the new asylum. The November wind had picked up, and it was getting dark. He had carefully gone over all the details of the building, thinking about the convenience of administering the building and the comfort and safety of its patients. All in all, the construction had been done in a substantial and thoughtful way using materials of good quality. He would write a listing of its impressive spaces to the trustees in his report of the results of his inspection and examination:

> To sum up: the whole building contains five hundred and forty-four rooms, (exclusive of closets) every room having one or more windows opening to the external air. There are twenty-four rooms in the front administration building for officers and apartments of officers; eighteen rooms in rear administration building for general dining-rooms, patients' reception parlors; amusement hall and chapel; six bath rooms and closets; five rooms in the kitchen department. In the rear buildings are twenty-six rooms for employes, thirteen for workshops, bakery and laundry purposes, and a boiler house. In the wings there are eighteen corridors, fifteen feet wide and from 140 feet to 175 feet long; two hundred and eighty-two single bedrooms for patients, and sixty-four associated dormitories; eighteen rooms for attendants or nurses; eighteen dining-rooms; eighteen parlors; and fifty-four rooms for bath rooms, lavatories and water closets—in all four hundred and fifty rooms in the wings.[27]

These are the facts of the design and construction of the asylum at Athens. Over the twenty years of the moral treatment experiment, adjustments and additions were made: two congregate dining rooms and rooms for seventy-two more patients in 1887,[28] stables and carriage house completed in 1876 and built anew in 1891 when the original burned, a coal house, a new straw house, a roof overhaul, new gutters, a new greenhouse, an icehouse, five electric lights installed as a trial in 1890, and the veranda. When Dr. Rutter returned as superintendent in 1880, he was clearly appalled at the physical state of the building and infrastructure, which had endured hard wear during the seven years after its completion. He enumerated the needs in his annual report to the trustees that year: the "foul and stagnant ponds in the bottoms east of the building which continue to emit their noxious vapors," the "grimy appearance of the walls in all but two of the wards," the heating apparatus which was "well-nigh worn out" and (because of the continual bursting of the hot water pipes) had "nearly ruined" the basement floors, the "inconvenience and utter unfitness" of the storeroom, the laundry machinery "so old and worn that it destroys a large amount of clothing besides failing to properly cleanse the remainder," and the necessity of an elevator to the fourth floor so that all patients might attend chapel services held there.[29] Dr. Rutter left the next year to become superintendent of the state asylum at Columbus, eighty miles away, leaving the list of refurbishments for new superintendent A. B. Richardson and steward R. E. Hamblin to accomplish.

Selections from *Views in and about Athens Asylum for the Insane: Picturesque Athens Asylum* (Columbus: Baker Photogravure Co., 1893). The entire volume, which was prepared for display at the 1893 World's Columbian Exposition in Chicago, may be viewed at http://media.library.ohiou.edu/. Images courtesy of the Athens County Historical Society and Museum, kindly loaned to Ohio University Libraries for digitizing and made available online by Ohio University Libraries.

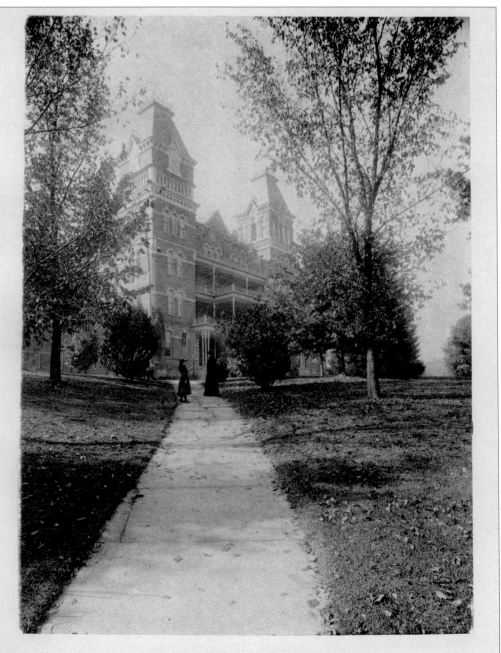

FRONT OF ADMINISTRATION BUILDING.

THE EAST ANGLE.

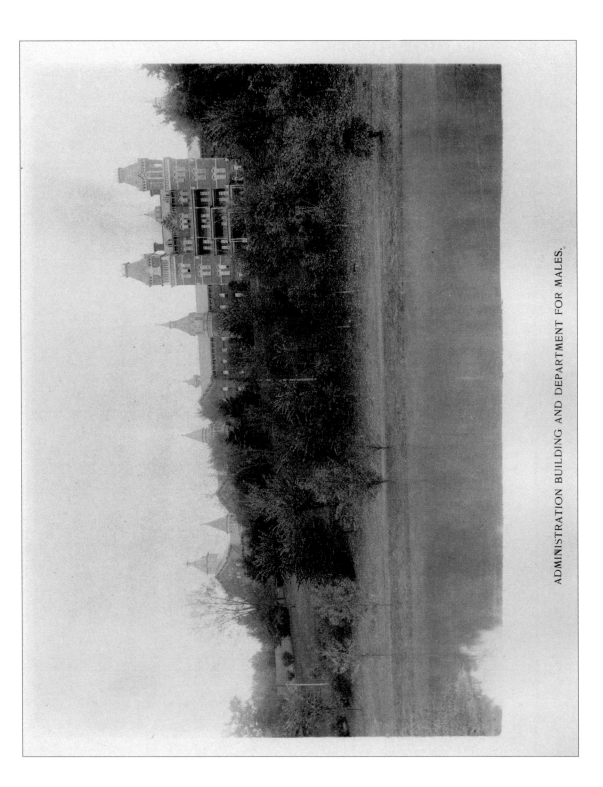

ADMINISTRATION BUILDING AND DEPARTMENT FOR MALES.

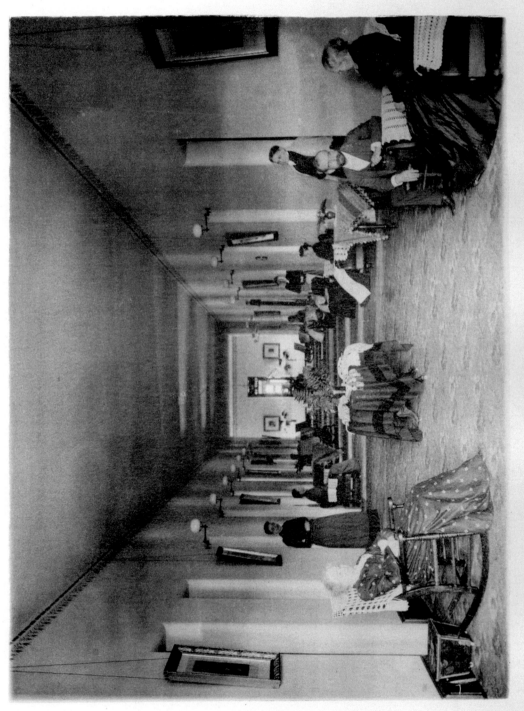

WARD FOR FEMALES.

WARD FOR MALES.

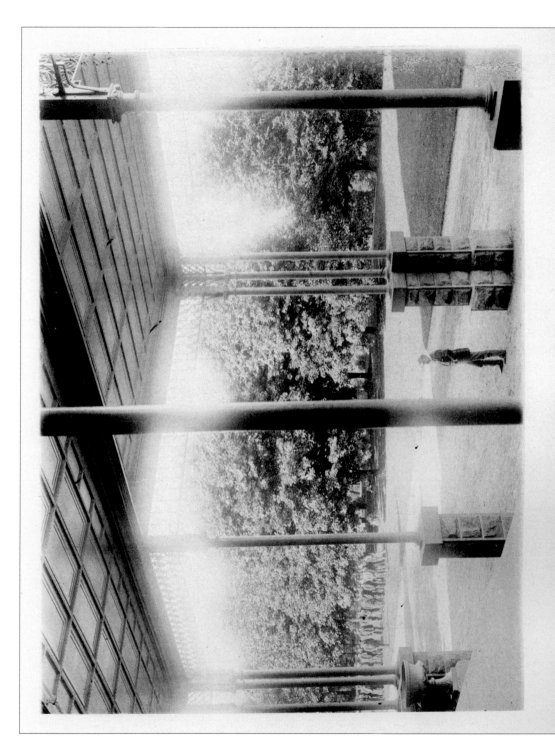

UNDER THE VERANDA.

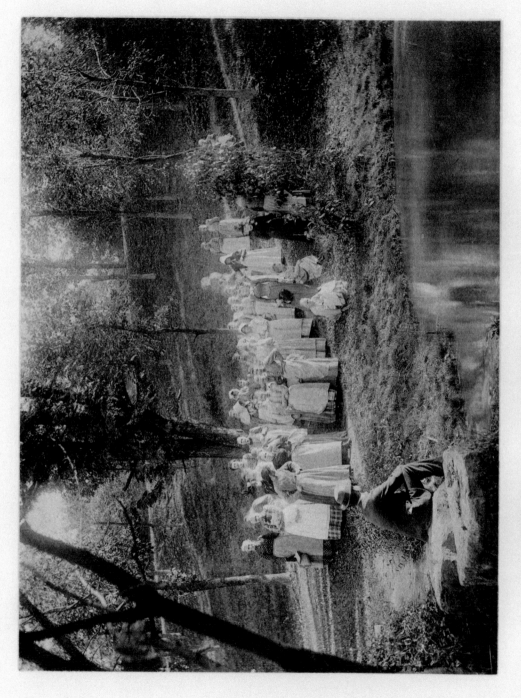

OUT FOR AN AIRING.

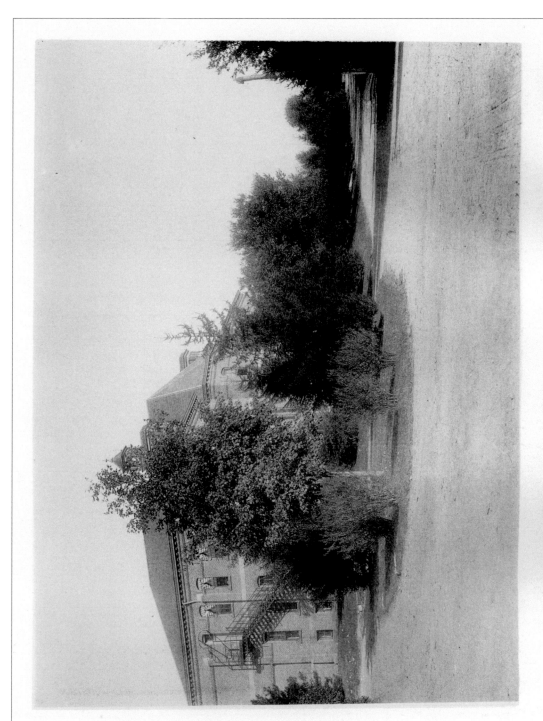

DEPARTMENT FOR MALES.   CONGREGATE DINING HALL AND WARD FOR INFIRM PATIENTS.

FROM THE NORTH-EAST.

VIEW OF WALK LEADING TOWARD TOWN.

THE LAKE.

APPROACH TO LOVER'S LANE.

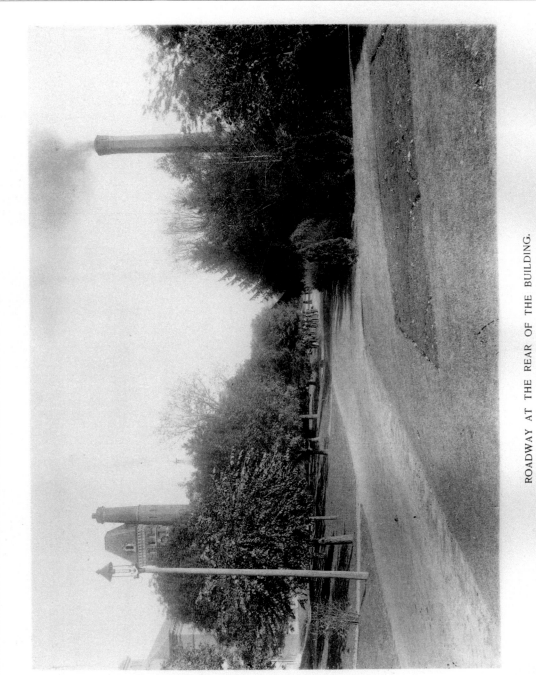

ROADWAY AT THE REAR OF THE BUILDING.

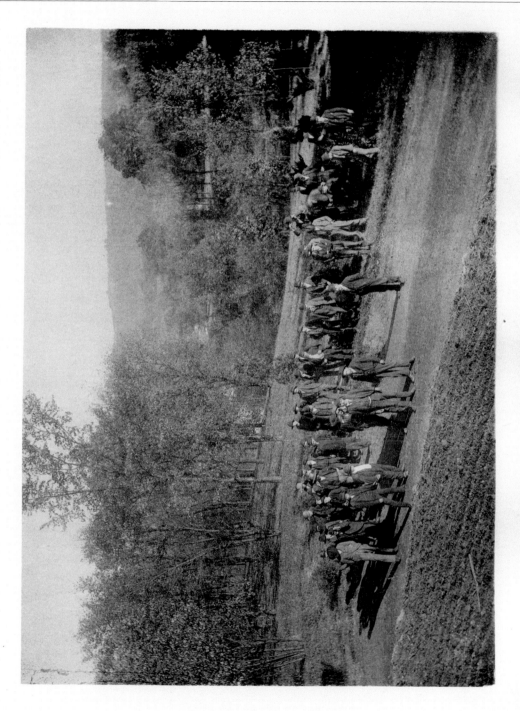

PATIENTS TAKING EXERCISE.

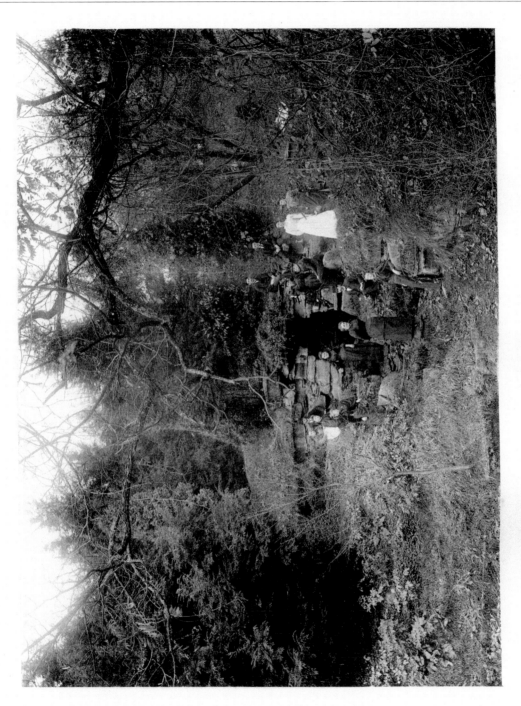

AT THE SPRING.

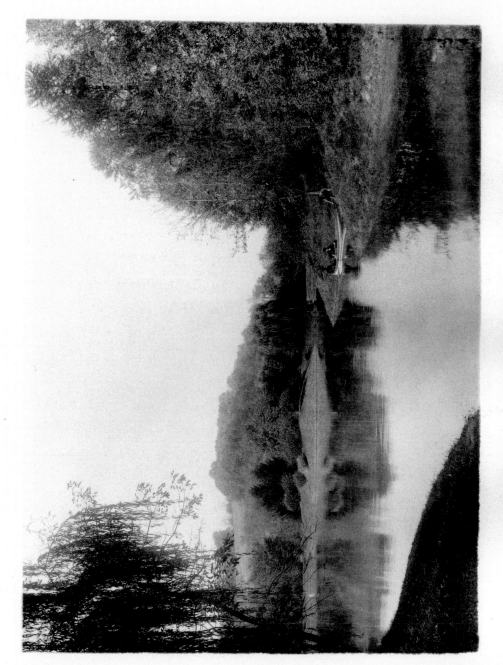

A LAKE VIEW WITH RESERVOIR HILL IN THE DISTANCE.

DRIFTING.

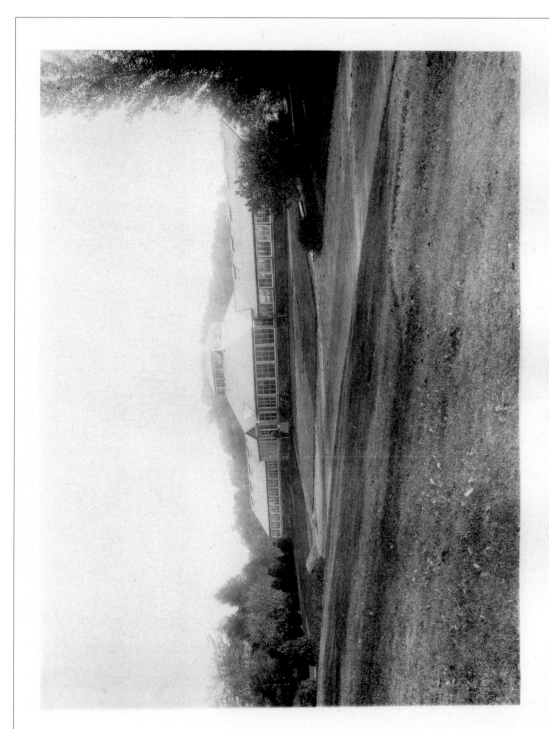

THE GREEN HOUSE.

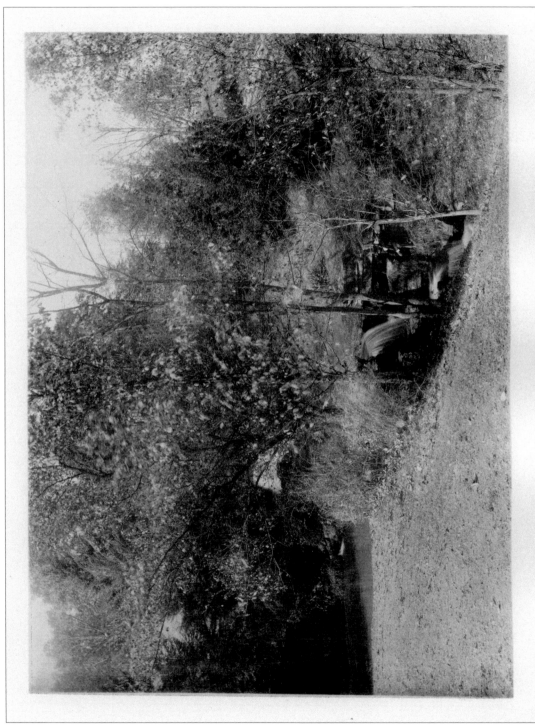

THE FALLS.

LOOKING NORTH-EAST FROM VERANDA.

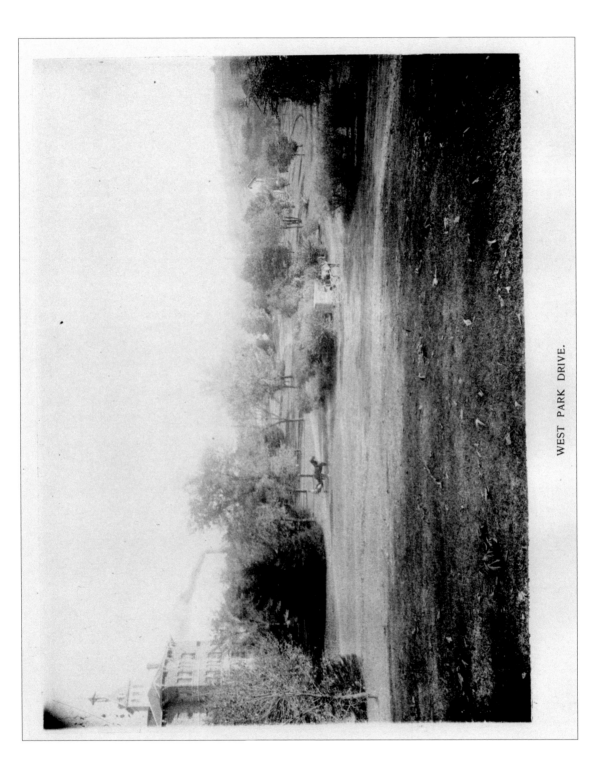

WEST PARK DRIVE.

FROM RESERVOIR HILL.

LOVER'S LANE.

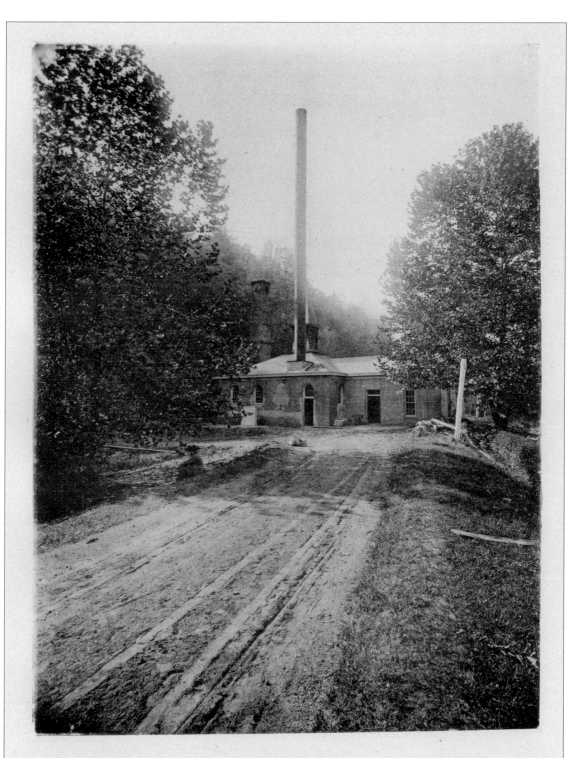

PUMP HOUSE.

POLITICS

"Partisan Interests and Personal Place-Seeking"

The State of Ohio's nineteenth-century commitment to free care for its citizens with mental illness resulted in a public investment in Athens to bricks and mortar, staff, families and patients, improvements, land acquisition, infrastructure, oversight, and research. Spending $621,000 in 1868 dollars[1] on a building embodying the moral treatment philosophy in the newly emerging field of psychiatry, staffing it at times with leading American alienists, and funding their proposals for innovations in care, the state-supported moral treatment experiment at Athens began under the leadership of Governor Rutherford B. Hayes and ended during the administration of Governor William McKinley. Both governors left office on being elected president of the United States, and each took his experience with the asylum at Athens with him.

Built during the post–Civil War years of industrial growth in Ohio, the asylum's first years were marked by the economic hardships of the Long Depression of 1873–79, a far-reaching economic calamity in which thousands of American businesses (both urban and rural) failed and unemployment reached 25 percent in some areas.[2] Through these grim economic troubles as well as the more prosperous times of the 1880s, the state government continued to pour money and political support into the asylum at Athens, demonstrating a commitment to providing care for Ohioans with mental illness as well as supporting its investment in bricks, mortar, purchasing and jobs. Patients and their families were expected to provide only clothing; beyond that, public asylum care in nineteenth-century Ohio was free. The state supported the entire operations of its asylums and paid for all aspects of patient care. Not until 1893, when the failure of banks and railroads led to another economic collapse, did the Board of State Charities propose that payment for care should be the responsibility of patients and families who could afford it. During times of economic contractions and struggles, the operations of the asylum at Athens were marked by tensions and problems produced in part by Ohio's political spoils system, known as reorganization. The years 1876–80 and 1891–93 saw turnover in trustees, superintendents, and staff. No new initiatives were undertaken except a fruitless and politically naïve quest for an asylum-based gas light plant; the emphasis during these times was on maintaining what had been built.

In contrast to the tensions that preceded and followed the decade of the 1880s, the asylum enjoyed the stability of nine years of leadership of Superintendent A. B. Richardson and Steward Robert E. Hamblin from 1881 through 1890. These men successfully negotiated the delicate nature of the reporting structure of steward and superintendent (the steward reported to both the trustees and the superintendent) and survived political party transitions in Columbus. Appointed by the board of trustees and reporting to both the trustees and the superintendent, the steward's dual reporting structure at times resulted in difficulties. The Ohio Board of State Charities reported to Ohio's governor in 1879 that the difficulties of the dual reporting line resulted in "a divided responsibility leading to a conflict of authority."[3] The most productive years of the moral treatment experiment were, in fact, during the tenures of three superintendents noted for their contributions to nineteenth-century psychiatry: Richard Gundry set the beginning course (1872–76), A. B. Richardson presided over a long period of harmony and innovation in treatment, and Henly Rutter stepped in for short periods between 1877 and 1880 to hold things together during political and staff turmoil. Consistent leadership was provided by Cincinnati-based landscape gardener Herman Haerlin and Athens landscaping contractor and gardener George Link, who spent his entire thirty-year career overseeing the execution of Haerlin's landscape plan. Ohio's governor and legislature supported the asylum's considerable grounds and landscaping infrastructure projects for its entire twenty years of moral treatment operations.

A century of asylum building in America preceded the 1868 groundbreaking for the asylum at Athens. Although the first public asylum in America was erected in Williamsburg, Virginia, in 1769, most eighteenth-century and early nineteenth-century American asylums were private. Quaker physicians and philanthropists in

Massachusetts, Pennsylvania, New York, and Connecticut began these private asylums, which featured an eclectic approach to treatment with such measures as warm baths, special diets, opium, force-feeding, bloodletting (at times), recreation, and employment at useful tasks. America's first public asylums opened in the South. The Western Lunatic Asylum in Staunton, Virginia, and the South Carolina Lunatic Asylum both opened in 1828.[4] These institutions admitted both affluent and poor patients and took a custodial orientation. In 1830 the Massachusetts legislature, prodded by education reformer and legislator Horace Mann, approved funding for Worcester State Hospital in Massachusetts, an asylum designed along the lines of moral treatment philosophy with the intention of providing curative and restorative care. Ohio followed, establishing the Ohio Lunatic Asylum at Columbus in 1835, which opened in 1838. The Pennsylvania Hospital for the Insane, a private asylum affiliated with the Pennsylvania Hospital in Philadelphia, opened in 1841 under the direction of Dr. Thomas Story Kirkbride.[5]

Massachusetts reformer Dorothea Dix stepped onto the national stage in the 1840s. She had traveled to England and learned there about moral treatment philosophy for mental illness during visits to the York Retreat founded by Quaker physician Samuel Tuke. She returned and successfully petitioned the Massachusetts legislature to expand its hospital at Worcester.[6] By the time Dix was forty years old, she had coped with a difficult and abusive childhood, suffered from continuing melancholia (a nineteenth-century term for various forms of depression), traveled in England and the United States, set herself up as a schoolteacher and prison reformer, and developed an astute political sense. Having decided to devote her life to improving conditions for those with mental illness, she became an unwavering political force.[7] Her method, beginning around 1840, was to travel to a state, conduct research and gather data on the plight of those with mental illness, present her findings to the state legislature, and persuade key politicians to support legislation to found a public asylum.[8] While visiting Columbus, Ohio, in the summer of 1846, Miss Dix became ill and stayed in Ohio to recover.[9]

In 1855, Ohio opened two more state asylums: the Northern Ohio Lunatic Asylum in Cleveland and the Southern Ohio Lunatic Asylum in Dayton. Four years later, the private Longview hospital in Cincinnati affiliated with the state of Ohio, so that Ohio then had four public asylums.[10] The Athens Lunatic Asylum, the fifth, was authorized by the Ohio legislature in 1867.

All five followed the architectural, landscape, organizational, and treatment tenets of the Kirkbride plan.

Ohio's state asylums were staffed and managed by a system of politics. The Athens Lunatic Asylum was governed by a board of trustees appointed by the governor, which included a "local" trustee from Athens to give the community a voice in hiring, purchasing, and other decision making. Post–Civil War Athens, a village of about 1,600 people, boasted a small mercantile community serving Ohio University.

But Athens lacked a cash-generating industry, the university's student enrollment was decreasing, and the university's trustees had failed to obtain legislative designation as a land-grant college, that having gone to Ohio State University in Columbus in 1866.[11] The asylum's payroll shored up cash flow in the village: the staff, most of whom lived on-site, crossed the bridge to town in Athens to shop for themselves and for the asylum. Local business concerns came to rely on the local trustee to represent their interests in obtaining contracts for goods and services. The asylum required a daily supply of coal, milk, meat, and natural gas, all purchased by contracts negotiated by its board of trustees. The contracts were nearly always awarded to Athens merchants and farmers. Coal, the contract for which was worth $6,000–$9,000 per year, went to companies based in Athens or nearby Nelsonville. The milk contract, negotiated every five years, was held by Athens dairy farmer James C. Bowers for over fifteen years. Meat, one of the largest line items in the asylum budget, was provided by an annual contract

FIGURE 4.1 Court Street in the village of Athens in the 1880s was lined with shops providing goods and services to the asylum. Court Street remained an earthen road, muddy in the rainy seasons, until 1893, when it became the first bricked street in Athens. Asylum employees lived on-site at the asylum and walked to town to visit the shops. The asylum steward purchased a vast array of goods and services from the town's merchants. *Courtesy of the Mahn Center for Archives and Special Collections, Ohio University Libraries.*

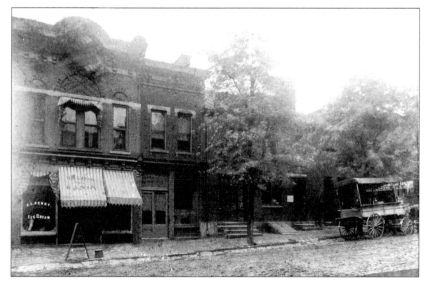

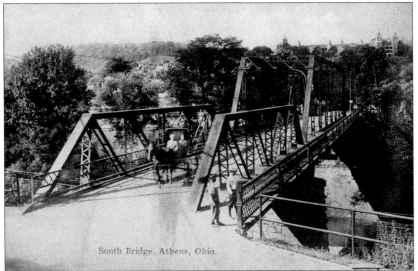

FIGURE 4.2 South Bridge over the Hocking River connected the asylum *(background)* with Athens. *Courtesy of the Mahn Center for Archives and Special Collections, Ohio University Libraries.*

with Athens meat market proprietor John Ring until 1882, when the asylum trustees decided to reduce the meat budget by bringing the butchering operation in-house.[12] The medical superintendent, in the nineteenth century a physician appointed by the board of trustees, oversaw the entire operation of the institution and assumed personal responsibility for the care of each patient.

TABLE 4.1

Medical superintendents of the Athens Lunatic Asylum, moral treatment era

Name	Years of service
Richard Gundry, MD	1872–76
Charles L. Wilson, MD	1877
Henly C. Rutter, MD	1877–78
P. H. Clarke, MD	1878–79
W. H. Holden, MD	1879–80
Henly C. Rutter, MD	1880–81
Alonzo B. Richardson, MD	1881–90
W. P. Crumbacker, MD	1890–92
C. O. Dunlap, MD	1892–96

Source: Board of Trustees of the Athens Asylum for the Insane, 1893 annual report, 614.

He nominated assistant physicians for appointment by the board, and the position of matron was filled by his wife. The superintendent was assisted by the steward, who hired attendants and other staff and oversaw all purchasing. Each year the steward prepared and submitted to the superintendent and the board of trustees a detailed report on everything he had purchased for the asylum and the monthly payrolls. The superintendent prepared a report for the trustees with a narrative summary of the year, sometimes expounding on treatment philosophy and recommendations, with many pages of statistics on admissions and treatment. The trustees added to these lengthy documents a short summary of contracts entered into (milk, beef, gas, coal, and land purchase), together with a budget request for the next year, and submitted the entire packet to the governor. The governor in turn packaged all this material with reports from other Ohio institutions and agencies, published the collected reports in several volumes, and submitted these volumes to the legislature. Overseeing the operations of all of Ohio's state charitable institutions and prisons was the Board of State Charities. The second state (after Massachusetts) to establish an oversight organization, Ohio set up its board in 1867, consisting of five members appointed by the governor. Although abolished soon after, it was reestablished in 1876 with Governor Rutherford B. Hayes as the ex-officio president. The Board of State Charities responded to complaints about the state's institutions and made inspections.[13]

Reorganization, the practice of replacing trustees and staff at Ohio's charitable institutions by a newly elected governor with a different political affiliation than the incumbent, was the mechanism by which the governor controlled leadership of state institutions. The Ohio Board of State Charities criticized the practice of reorganization for decades before it was finally abolished in the twentieth century. In 1880, the board complained that most of the "cruelties and irregularities of state charitable institutions were because "partisan politics had crept into them and disturbed their administration."[14] The board's secretary explained how political appointments led to bad hiring practices from the medical superintendent to ward attendants:

> Often local parties . . . aspire to the control of appointments,
> first of Trustees, and through these of subordinates.
> Oftentimes individuals, aspiring to places, select an
> intelligent, honest, unaspiring citizen, such an one as
> would surely command the confidence and respect of the
> [Governor], and bring his name forward as a suitable person,
> and secure his appointment as a Trustee of one of our
> benevolent institutions. Having secured the appointment,

the next step is a comparatively easy one—that is, to urge personal claims upon such Trustee to an appointment in the institution over which he may have been appointed. Such manipulation is carried forward more or less successfully at every reorganizing period, and in such manner as that neither the Governor nor his appointee may suspect that even partisan interests, much less personal place-seeking, has been the ruling motive. . . . [B]y these and kindred methods the doors of our institutions are thrown open to unworthy persons . . . and our entire system of public benevolence brought into discredit.[15]

The asylum was founded, built, and opened under a series of Republican governors.

TABLE 4.2
Ohio governors, 1866–96

Governor	Term	Political party
Jacob D. Cox	1866–68	Republican
Rutherford B. Hayes	1868–72	Republican
Edward F. Noyes	1872–74	Republican
William Allen	1874–76	Democratic
Rutherford B. Hayes	1876–77	Republican
Thomas L. Young	1877–78	Republican
Richard M. Bishop	1878–80	Democratic
Charles Foster	1880–84	Republican
George Hoadly	1884–86	Democratic
Joseph B. Foraker	1886–90	Republican
James E. Campbell	1890–92	Democratic
William McKinley	1892–96	Republican

Source: Ohio Historical Society Editors, *The Governors of Ohio*, 2nd ed. (Columbus: Ohio Historical Society, 1969). Ohio's governors served two-year terms until 1957, when the term was changed to four years.

Governor Rutherford B. Hayes oversaw the construction of the new asylum and appointed its first medical superintendent, tapping Dr. Richard H. Gundry for the post in 1872. Governor Hayes remained close with Superintendent Gundry, visiting him in 1875 at the asylum as Hayes campaigned for his second term as Ohio's governor, making there what he described as a "sober, strong, but dull speech."[16] Upon election to his second term as governor in 1876, Hayes worked through the trustees of the state's

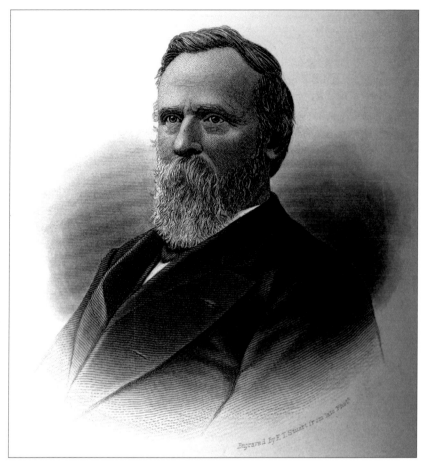

asylum at Columbus to appoint Gundry medical superintendent there. Ever political, in a note to the editor of the *Cleveland Leader* about his prospects for the upcoming presidential election, Hayes ended with a postscript about the asylum appointments: "I am very glad the asylum appointments are satisfactory."[17] Soon after, in 1877, Hayes's political career took him to Washington as president. At Gundry's death in 1891 while superintendent of Spring Grove Asylum in Maryland, Hayes wrote in his journal that he "received a dispatch . . . of the death of . . . Richard Gundry. He was formerly in charge of the lunatic asylum at Dayton, afterwards at Athens. A very able, wise, and skilful man in his profession, and of large general ability and culture. I sent a dispatch of condolence and appreciation. He was one of the friends made in public life, when I was governor of Ohio."[18]

Hayes was deeply familiar with asylums and care for those with mental illness. As a young Cincinnati lawyer, he had been the court-appointed lawyer for the jury trial of Nancy Farrer, in which he obtained a verdict of guilty by way of insanity. Hayes noted with satisfaction in his journal that "she will now go to a lunatic asylum, and so my first case involving life is ended successfully."[19] Closer to home, Dr. Joseph T. Webb, brother of Governor Hayes's wife, Lucy Webb Hayes, was appointed superintendent of Longview Asylum at Cincinnati in 1871. In a letter to his uncle, Hayes enthusiastically described the benefits of his brother-in-law's new position and noted that Dr. Webb had received the appointment without the help of the governor's office. Longview at the time was a locally run asylum, with only partial participation from state government, and its trustees surely must have thought it advantageous to have the governor's brother-in-law as its medical superintendent. Dr. Webb for his part must have found the steady work and substantial benefits attractive.

> You have perhaps noticed that Doctor Joe has been appointed the Superintendent of the Longview Asylum. I am glad of it. It is altogether the best position for a physician in Ohio. It is a county and city affair, with a partial control in the State. The place is more permanent and better paid than anything else of the sort we have. Being under a board of city men they are liberal in all respects. The pay is thirty-five hundred dollars, and the officer is allowed absolutely everything but his clothing— servants, carriage, and horses, house rent, and living all complete. The only drawback is health, and the doctor thinks he can make that what it should be. He got it [the appointment] without pushing and without [me] interfering. I did not know of it.[20]

Hayes was familiar with asylum life, as he and his family often visited Dr. Webb at Longview, spending the Fourth of July holiday there in 1872. A few months later he visited and described the landscape there to his uncle: "We came out to spend Sunday with Uncle Joe and go back Monday. We are all well. . . . I have been looking at some of the doctor's vines on walls and trees. The Virginia creeper, the Chinese wistaria [sic] and the English ivy soon make an old tree a beautiful object."[21]

Hayes's other brother-in-law, Dr. James D. Webb, became a patient at this asylum and died there in 1873. Hayes wrote his son Webb of the news: "We have just heard of the death of your Uncle, Dr. James D. Webb, at Carthage, in the asylum. He has been gradually growing worse for several weeks. We shall go . . . down to the funeral tomorrow. It is a sad termination of his life, but after we knew that there was organic disease of the brain, it has been the only possible result."[22]

Governor Hayes's friend Dr. Gundry departed Athens in 1876 to lead the asylum in Ohio's capital at Columbus, and the Athens trustees appointed Indianapolis resident Dr. Charles Wilson in his stead. Wilson had practiced medicine in the Athens area before he left for Indiana. Caught in a "blistering crossfire of statewide, partisan politicking ostensibly about his non-resident status," Wilson served for less than a month and returned to Indiana.[23] Henly Rutter, a Republican, was elected by the trustees in Wilson's stead. During his tenure (1877–78), Dr. Rutter enlarged the kitchen garden, secured funding from the state to substitute new six-inch water mains for the three-inch ones, began construction on a reservoir, built a coalhouse, and asked for a veranda to protect the front entrance. Rutter resigned at the election of Democratic governor Richard Bishop, moved to Cincinnati to practice medicine, and wrote a paper on epilepsy for the Board of State Charities.[24]

Reorganization repeatedly affected leadership at the asylum at Athens. Following the election of Bishop as governor in 1878, all the trustees and officers were replaced. That year and the next (1879), the attention of Athens as well as the state media was riveted upon rumors and complaints about Democratic appointee Superintendent P. H. Clarke, who served for only one year. The Board of State Charities, with tactful circumspection, referred to the departure of Clarke and his staff for reasons unknown: "The disturbances leading to the change in the entire medical staff of this asylum are not definitely known."[25] Assistant physicians Joseph Hanley and Josiah Lash were dismissed from the asylum, whereupon they wrote a letter of complaint about Superintendent Clarke and the trustees to the Ohio legislature.

> To the Honorable House of Representatives of the
> General Assembly of the State of Ohio:
>
> We humbly pray your honorable body to support the
> resolution of representative Charles Townsend of this
> county asking that a committee of your members be
> appointed to investigate the management of the Athens
> Asylum for the Insane.

We consider that the so-called investigation by the trustees, on the 17th day of april 1879 was incomplete, and that its decision was unjust and wrong.

In support of our plea for an investigation, we emphatically allege that Dr. P[leasant] H[enry] Clarke is incompetent and totally unfit to fill the responsible position of superintendent of such institution. As specifications we allege that he is heedless, careless, and inattentive to the true and proper interests of the unfortunates therein confined; that he wholly fails to enforce discipline among either patients or employees; that he habitually absents himself from his office and proper place of business, and shuts himself up for hours at a time where he cannot be found, and fails to visit the wards as often as a superintendent should; that during the absence from the building, on leave, of the assistant physician on the female side of the house while those wards were under his [Clarke's] charge, he neglected for three days, although frequently requested to do so by the attendant, to visit and properly administer to the wants of a sick patient and that within a day or two thereafter she died; that he is habitually addicted to the immoderate use of opium and intoxicating drinks, that he has frequently been found in his private office in a drunken stupor or sleep, with a bottle of intoxicating drink on a table by his side; that he has been found beastly drunk in his private office at the unseasonable hour of two o'clock at night; that he has been known to take beer bottles from the storage drug room late at night to his bed chamber, and that they have been carried out of there by the chamber maid in the morning; that he continually kept in his private office a bottle of whisky; that he has frequently gone into the wards in a stupid and staggering condition, his breath smelling of whisky; that he has been unable to prescribe for patients when he has been sent off to see them, and often went away without doing so, that, in fact, his stupid and intemperate habits are generally understood and talked about among the attendants and employees in the building and that the effect is demoralizing and degrading. We further allege that the Board of Trustees of the Athens Asylum for the Insane has been for months cognizant of the character and habits of Dr. P.H. Clarke, its superintendent, and that until very recently they persistently refused and failed to give it any attention; that certain ones of them have been accustomed to drink with the superintendent when they visited the building, and have been seen at different times and late at night in a drunken condition with him, and that their rooms in the morning have exhibited striking evidences of the previous night's debauch. In substantiation of what we here declare, we beg leave to refer to the evidence of parties as familiar with these facts as we are ourselves which is hereto attached and made a part of this memorial.

Respectfully submitted,
J[oseph] M. HANLEY, M.D.
J[osiah] W[ilson] LASH, M.D.
Late Assistant Physicians of the Athens Asylum for Insane
Athens, O., April 21st, 1879
Subscribed and sworn to before me this 21st day of April,
   A.D., 1879,
George W. Baker, Clerk, Common Pleas Court, Athens
   Co., O.[26]

In Athens in 1879, rumors of opium eating and drunkenness swirled. The letters written back and forth among members of the Zenner family of Athens provide insight into the community's perspective. Originally from Cincinnati, the Zenners wrote often to Phillip Zenner, who was in Europe studying medicine. In April 1879, Phillip's brother-in-law John Friday wrote that "there was big trouble over at the asylum, the trustees had Dr. Clarke on trial for opium eating and drunkenness, charge by Drs. Hanley and Lash, the consequence was, they threw [out] or discharged the two latter physicians and a great many attendants. All quiet again."[27] Two months later, Friday wrote again to Phillip, attributing the unfolding scandal to politics and jealousy: "[T]here has been a great change in the Asylum here. A great deal of scandal has been generally circulated. Much of it however is due to potential jealousys and bickering. Clarke the supt. resigned his position and Dr. Holden from Zanesville was elected in his stead. Also Drs. Hanley and Lash were thrown out of their positions and new assistant physicians appointed."[28] Phillip's brother Henry likewise wrote to him: "They have been having a big fuss over at the asylum. Dr. Hanley and Lash have been discharged and also the druggist Ellis and quite a number of the ward attendants have also left. Clarke has been accused of drunkenness by the most of those discharged, and great efforts are being made to obtain his removal on the grounds of total inability for the management of the concern."[29] David Zenner, the head of the family, put the matter into the context of local affairs: "Athens is the same as ever. The new courthouse is rising out of the pavement. Townfolks [are occupied with] politics and scold at the Asylum and farmers grumble at the weather and the scarcity of money, but 'among us' if their apple trees instead of apple blossoms would bear five dollar bills they would grumble still at their not being of higher denomination."[30]

A close reading of Dr. Clarke's 1879 report to the trustees suggests that Dr. Clarke introduced measures and criticisms that were likely unpopular among staff, patients, trustees, and the community First, he reduced tobacco consumption among patients and staff from 250 to 20 pounds per month. Second, he eliminated alcohol rations to patients. Third, he was extremely disapproving of the conditions he found at the asylum. He criticized the library ("entirely too small"), the grounds in front of the male wards ("very ragged and repulsive"), the wards ("gloomy and dungeon-like"), the supply of surgical instruments ("deficient"), the refrigerator for preserving meats and milk ("partly decayed"), the straw-house ("entirely too small"), and the propagating house ("rotten and unsafe").[31] Finally, Dr. Clarke had the politically ill-conceived idea to cancel the asylum's contract with the Athens Gas Light Company and adopt electric lighting. While electricity was the latest thing in lighting, the asylum was also the single largest customer of the Athens-based gas company, and a canceled contract would no doubt have been disastrous for that Athens business establishment.[32]

Yet another problem developed at the asylum. Abuse of patients by attendants prompted an investigation by the Board of State Charities. The secretary of the board visited Athens to inspect the asylum and wrote of the abuse of patients that he witnessed there.

> Twice since the [1879] reorganization I witnessed, in
> person, violent treatment of patients. On one occasion
> I saw there attendants attempting by force, to remove a
> patient from one ward to another. They were all stout
> men. . . . [T]hese three men had thrown the patient

violently upon the floor—I heard the scuffle and the fall and went into the ward—the three were holding the patient, two at his feet to prevent his kicking, the other one was choking him. . . . [O]n another occasion I witnessed a most unprovoked and unpardonable treatment of an apparently quiet and inoffensive patient by a swaggering, overgrown bully employed as an attendant. The Catholic priest, of Athens, and Dr. Hanley, one of the Assistant Physicians, were present at the time when this ruffian seized the patient rudely by the collar, and jerked him violently from his seat, and shook him with fearful force. . . . [F]eeling incensed at this display of brutality, I asked the attendant why he treated the patient in this manner. His reply indicated the brute more than his violence, it was simply this, "he had no business to sit down there." Dr. Hanley was the physician to the female wards; he was not responsible for the treatment of male patients; he dared not interfere, he did all he could do; he informed Dr. Lash, Assistant Physician in male wards, of what had occurred. Dr. Lash inquired for the particular[s], I gave them to him, knowing that he, too, had no authority in such cases. At the earliest opportunity I communicated the facts to one of the Trustees, Dr. Ball, who said that he was glad to have his attention called to these facts, and that he would see to the prompt dismissal of the attendant.[33]

Both Dr. Hanley and Dr. Lash were dismissed, and the controversial Dr. Clarke was replaced by Dr. W. H. Holden. But matters only worsened. The Ohio legislature accused the Athens asylum of financial mismanagement and launched an investigation. Summarizing the asylum's litany of troubles, the local newspaper reported on the headlines around the state critical of the asylum.

The result of the visit here . . . of the House Committee on Finance has been to supply the daily press with articles crowned with startling head lines and in which are detailed instances of alleged gross financial mismanagement of the Hospital for the Insane here, specifying . . . that the institution . . . cost last year $136,547.66, while there is a deficiency bill of over $15,000, that the estimate for this year contemplates something over $179,000, that the committee inquired into the payroll, and learned that it exceeds $2,000 per month, exclusive of officers' salaries, and that Superintendent Holden admitted that it is much larger than the pay roll for the Dayton Asylum, an institution with no greater number of inmates. Another editor is informed by a member of the committee that the whole institution is in a woeful condition, that the expenses have been run about $25,000 beyond the appropriation . . . that Steward Bell kept one account and the Superintendent another, that they do not at all correspond, and finally that the committee are of the opinion that there has been general extravagance.[34]

Then a patient died, allegedly at the hands of attendants. The Board of State Charities investigated, and though the investigation fell short of confirming the allegation, the board acknowledged its essential truth: "That a patient was fatally beaten in the Athens Asylum, is asserted by patients, and the present Superintendent, I know, entertains grave apprehension of its truth by an attendant in the Athens Asylum. It is asserted by patients and Superintendent that he had been dismissed already for lesser wrongs. . . . [T]he persons perpetrating the great wrong had been dismissed for lesser causes before the facts of the greater became known."[35]

Despite the allegations of murder and fiscal mismanagement, the state continued to respond to requests from the Athens trustees, providing additional appropriations for fire hoses, levee and reservoir building, and road construction. The trustees were happy to report to the governor the "exercising of strict economy in every department" for the year 1878 so that "a large sum of money" might be saved for the state.[36] The following year, however, Superintendent Holden complained about the condition of the physical plant of the asylum as well as the "entirely inadequate" state allocation of two thousand dollars for grading and road building. Newly elected Republican governor Charles Foster then appointed a new board of trustees, which promptly replaced Superintendent Holden with Dr. Henly C. Rutter. The asylum management regained its equilibrium. Rutter, a Republican, and his steward, Democrat R. E. Hamblin, were welcomed back by the community. Even the village's Republican newspaper, which grumbled at Hamblin's appointment, grudgingly acknowledged his skills and fitness for the job and noted that "to see the once familiar faces of . . . Rutter and . . . Hamblin around on our streets once more calls up pleasant associations of olden time."[37]

To honor Rutter's return, a patient at the asylum composed a long poem commenting on the problems of reorganization, politics, money, and patient abuse that had plagued the asylum and engaged the community. He intended to mail the poem to a friend, but it was filed away instead with the new superintendent's correspondence. The poet, who called himself Rat Trap Man, was a prolific writer of verse and prose in both English and German; his literary efforts were kept in the asylum's files of superintendent correspondence. The poet ends with his hope that alcohol service would be restored to patients.

I have some quacks, I will tell them by name,
But remember, none of them, ever had name . . .
Holden, Eddy, Rallston, Hallson & Dr. Ball
As Experts, & Outlaws, their equals can not be found at all.
In no country, upon the entire globe,
But their time of Justice is near, I hope.
Of Holden I could fill an Enquirer's triple sheet.
But the Law of Ohio, will send him where they don't sow any wheat.
I have a Loonatic Asylum, called *charity* institution,
And in fact, it *must* undergo a great revolution.
For while Holden was boss, the inmates were shamefully treated,
And by the attendants, kicked, struck[,] chucked and beated.
But Solomon said, there is a time for all.
A time for sorrow and pleasure, & a time to go to the Ball.
There was also a time, when democratic thieves plundered this state,
But Honest Republicans took charge of it, of late.
Calico charley, was elected chief magistrate,
And he kicked a good many democratic thieves through the gate.
Scoundral Holden was kicked out,
         And Dr. Rutter put in his place
That Holden is an Outlaw, & that
         Dr. Rutter a man of honor you
Can read in their face!
The wind blows quite different, Since Dr. Rutter, is boss.
And, I think, US, taxpayers want be as much, at Loss.
To reduce expenses, is what he has on his Brain.
And I have for the last year, seeker for liberty but in vain.
But the old says is, live in Hopes, & you will never be in despair.
And Dr. Rutter, told me, he will do, what is fair.
Therefore I think, the day is very near,

That I can have, as heretofore my quantum of lagerbeer.
Now my best respects to all the boys in blue.
Coming election, I'll sound for the Democrats, a tattoo.
    (Lights out!)[38]

Dr. Rutter did indeed reduce expenses, eliminating thirty-nine persons from the annual payroll and reducing gas consumption. The local paper described this in vivid terms: "[R]eform in the Athens Asylum is illustrated in the fact that Dr. Rutter found forty more paid employees hanging on the ragged edge of the institution on his return there than when he left two years ago. . . . These supernumeraries were . . . unceremoniously bounced at the beginning of the week."[39] The state provided Dr. Rutter and the trustees extra funds to repaint the building's exterior woodwork and towers, enlarge the straw-house, and purchase new pictures for the wards. Newly elected governor Charles Foster (the "Calico Charley" referred to by Rat Trap Man in his poem) took the unusual step of visiting the asylum monthly to check on operations.

When Rutter was called to the superintendent's post at the Columbus asylum in 1881, Dr. A. B. Richardson was appointed by the trustees to fill his place. The management team of Superintendent Richardson and Steward R. E. Hamblin remained in place through seven years of Republican governors as well as Democratic governor George Hoadly's 1884–86 term.[40] Dr. Richardson and the trustees asked governors for funds over and above regular operating costs to improve the building and its landscape, arguing for the essential curative nature of beautiful views and orderly, attractive surroundings. The state sent funds to enlarge the system of lakes, "tastefully frescoe" the amusement hall, purchase new pictures for the wards, repaint the interior spaces, replace furniture, pay for many acres of landscaping, and enlarge the conservatory and replace all its glass. To shore up the institution's infrastructure, the state provided money to install a new stone floor in the laundry, install a telephone line to a pharmacy in Athens, replace all the gutters, enlarge pipes carrying the steam heat (the old ones produced a pounding noise, which was a constant source of annoyance to all), build a new icehouse, repaint the billiards room, build a wagon shed, construct a road in Athens from the bridge to the railroad station, and build a seven-foot-wide stone path from the asylum to the bridge that led to town. Finally, the state appropriated funds to pay for the construction of two patient congregate dining rooms, the first in an American public asylum; add rooms for 150 patients above the dining rooms; and hire an additional assistant physician to care for the growing number of patients. The trustees also approved the hiring of the nation's first female asylum physician, Dr. Agnes Johnson. These projects were paid for by the state in amounts over and above the asylum's usual annual operating budget.[41]

Dr. Richardson did not keep his position beyond the election of Democratic governor James E. Campbell in 1890. He may have seen the political handwriting on the wall with his critique of political reorganization in his 1889 annual report, where he wrote that "science suffers when medical officers are required to take into account meeting the wishes of party managers."[42] That year, two of his assistant physicians, Dr. Agnes Johnson and Dr. Crumbacker, were removed; the following year, Richardson was replaced by Dr. Crumbacker.

Republican governor William McKinley oversaw the last years of the moral treatment experiment at Athens. Upon his election as governor in 1892, he replaced the entire professional staff installed by Democratic governor Campbell at Athens. On McKinley's watch, new boilers were installed, additional land was purchased for the vegetable garden, the asylum's amusement hall was converted to sleeping quarters for staff, and an abundance of ice was harvested from the asylum's lakes to cool the drinking water of patients and staff during the summer. Governor McKinley also provided funds to construct the long-requested veranda over the asylum entrance. The resources of all state institutions were marshaled by the governor's administration to provide exhibits at the 1893 World's Columbian Exposition at Chicago, and the Athens asylum sent photographs of its grounds and building as well as "numerous articles of fancy work" made by patients."[43] (Coincidentally, nine years later at the Pan-American Exposition at Buffalo, President McKinley, while making a speech, was assassinated by a man who, it was later argued, belonged in an insane asylum.)

McKinley was instrumental in establishing Massillon State Hospital in northeastern Ohio. Moral treatment as a philosophical and architectural model for treating mental illness began to give way to a new model known as the "cottage plan," and Massillon was one of the first in the nation to be built along these therapeutic lines. Even while coping with prolonged industrial depression and unemployment set off by the Panic of 1893, McKinley devoted energy to securing a donation of 240 acres for the new

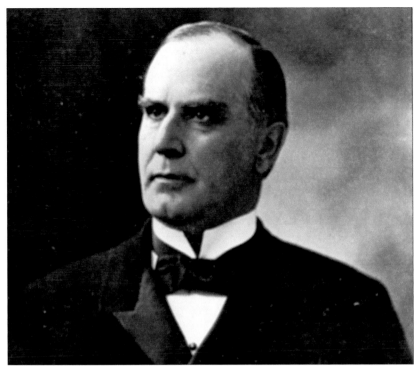

state hospital for persons with mental illness, and he tapped former Athens superintendent A. B. Richardson as a member of its
board of construction and later its first superintendent. In 1899, his
second year in office, President McKinley appointed alienist Richardson to the prestigious post in Washington of superintendent
at Saint Elizabeths Government Hospital for the Insane.[44] Saint
Elizabeths was founded in 1855 by mental health reformer Dorothea Dix as the Government Hospital for the Insane to provide for
the mental health needs of members of the U.S. Army and Navy as
well as residents of the District of Columbia.[45] At its peak population, Saint Elizabeths housed seven thousand patients. McKinley needed a superintendent who could improve and enlarge the
building, its landscape, and its infrastructure while supervising the
provision of care. On his appointment, Dr. Richardson astounded
Washington and the asylum community by immediately securing
a congressional appropriation, by unanimous vote in the House
of Representatives, of a million dollars for twelve new buildings,
the construction of which he personally supervised. He became a
part of Washington's medical elite, being invited to join the prestigious Cosmos Club, and was elected chair of the department of
mental diseases at Columbian Medical School (now Georgetown
University). Just a few weeks before his death in 1903, Richardson

was elected president of the American Medico-Psychological Association, the forerunner of the American Psychiatric Association. Dr. Richardson collapsed at work from apoplexy and died within a few hours at the age of fifty-one. Colleagues who eulogized him described his nature as strong, determined, convivial, earnest, and thoughtful and his life as an "uninterrupted series of successes."[46]

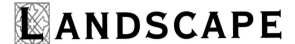ANDSCAPE

"Of Beautiful and Varied Scenery"

T he landscape of the Athens Lunatic Asylum was a product of climate change, the religious and psychological
significance attributed by Native Americans to the site, careful
planning by German-born Cincinnati landscape designer Herman Haerlin, the life work of groundsman and landscaper George
Link, the asylum's trustees and superintendents, Ohio's lawmak-
ers who allocated funds to attend to the landscape, and the toil
of male asylum patients as well as that of Athens townsmen who
graded, smoothed, and planted the steeply terraced land. The site
for the Athens Lunatic Asylum, which eventually encompassed
over a thousand acres, began with 150 acres of steep hills and
meadows on a terrace high above the Hocking River. Superintendent Richard Gundry, in a report to the board of trustees during
construction of the hospital, wrote that the site was "admirably
adapted to the purposes of the landscape gardener, to develop the
pleasure-grounds and gardens, drives and walks, of such interest to all, but so necessary for the comfort of those who may be
compelled to spend months or years, or even pass away the rest of
their lives within its boundaries."[1]

The terraces of the site were rugged and steep, created by glacial outwash pushed into the river. Their topography is obvious
even today in the forests between the river and asylum buildings.
In the nineteenth century, the citizens of Athens had a fine view of
the asylum site and watched the asylum, a symbol of the community's hopes for both mental healing and economic gain, take shape
across the river. Merchant John Ballard wrote to his son in January 1869 of the progress of construction. As the building became
visible, Ballard noted the altered landscape. "The New Lunatic

Assylum [*sic*] will make quite an imposing appearance from this Village. The Sycamore Grove just over the river is all demolished."[2]

A beautiful and highly developed landscape was axiomatic to moral treatment philosophy, and the landscape developed at Athens was second to none. Groves of trees, attractive scenery, and handsomely cultivated land functioned as attractive vistas on which patients could gaze, sites for patient work and exercise, a place for farming operations, and an inviting reassurance to families and patients. From the beginning, the asylum's trustees were committed to developing a beautiful and curative landscape. They included in their annual report to the governor the superintendent's request for funds to continue grounds improvements, "that our poor unfortunates who are necessarily confined in the wards may look out upon a landscape with pleasure and delight."[3]

The asylum's grounds were designed in 1867 by Cincinnati landscape gardener Herman Haerlin, whose design sensibility was rooted in Frederick Law Olmsted's vision of the recuperative power of authentic natural landscapes and preservation of original wilderness.[4] Olmsted planned the grounds for several asylums, including Buffalo State Hospital (completed in 1895), Hudson River State Hospital (1871), and McLean Hospital, the private state mental hospital in Boston in which he died in 1903. Haerlin began his career as a greenhouse proprietor in Cincinnati; the landscape design of the Athens asylum was his first major commission. After

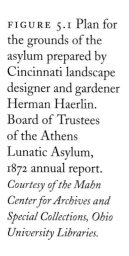

FIGURE 5.1 Plan for the grounds of the asylum prepared by Cincinnati landscape designer and gardener Herman Haerlin. Board of Trustees of the Athens Lunatic Asylum, 1872 annual report. *Courtesy of the Mahn Center for Archives and Special Collections, Ohio University Libraries.*

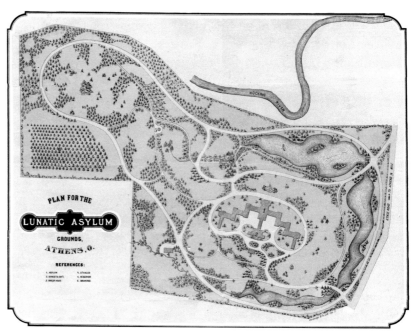

the success of this project, he went on to design the campus plan for Ohio State University and urban parks in Chillicothe, Springfield, and other Ohio cities. Haerlin ended his career as chief gardener at the new National Military Home in Springfield, Ohio. A distinguished-looking man with a Teddy Roosevelt–style moustache, a square jaw, and serious eyes, Haerlin was experienced in a wide array of civic and political affairs. Ohio's governor appointed him state commissioner in charge of the vast floral exhibition and competition at Ohio's 1888 Centennial Fair in Columbus.[5] Occasionally he was called upon to serve as an expert witness in judicial cases involving horticultural matters, such as one in which he was asked to estimate the value of a sycamore tree that had been cut down to make way for a Cincinnati trolley line.

Yet Haerlin was foremost a gardener and garden designer, all through his career developing meticulous plans for civic parks that remain today graceful natural landscapes, centerpieces of beauty for Ohio's towns and university campuses. With a careful eye for detail, Haerlin personally supervised the development of his landscapes. His plan for the landscape of the Athens Lunatic Asylum was adopted by its board of trustees in 1868, yet he continued visiting the asylum at Athens for another fifteen years to supervise details, from planting flowers to developing plans for sewage treatment to personally selecting and transporting evergreen seedlings to the asylum and providing clean water for patients and staff. For years the asylum superintendents, in their annual reports to the trustees, wrote of the importance and excellence of Haerlin's work in moving forward the landscape plans and projects. Wrote the superintendent in 1876, for example, "Our flower

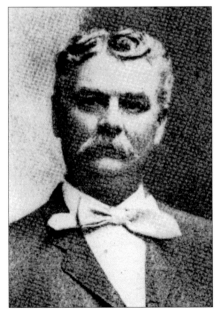

FIGURE 5.2 Herman Haerlin, Cincinnati landscape designer and gardener. Haerlin designed the landscape plan for the asylum, which was executed by George Link, gardener and landscaping supervisor at the asylum 1871–1903. Originally published in "Herman Haerlin," *Gardening* 14 (1906): 354. *Image provided by the Chicago Public Library.*

gardens and green-house have been very successfully cultivated and have yielded pleasure to all sensible of the charms of nature. That part of the grounds already finished attests the skill and taste of the landscape gardener, Mr. Haerlin, and wins the admiration of all beholders."[6] The asylum's leadership, with money allocated by Governor Rutherford B. Hayes and the design expertise and vision of Mr. Haerlin, early on accomplished two goals for the asylum's infrastructure: providing filtered drinking water and beginning a successful gardening operation. For its first five years of operations, the asylum obtained water directly from the Hocking River by means of pipes and pumps, without benefit of a filtration system. A modest river, just a trickle compared to the Ohio River into which it flowed thirty miles away, the Hocking is often muddy. Dr. Richard Gundry, in his annual report to Ohio's Governor Rutherford B. Hayes, described this chocolate-colored drinking water:

> I beg to call your attention to some facts connected with the supply of water to the Hospital. It is pumped from the Hocking River into a reservoir on the top of a hill somewhat higher than the roof of the house. The water is soft and the supply ample, but whenever a freshet occurs, or even after a heavy shower, the stream becomes very turbid and the water is muddy and discolored. Yet such we must use or have none. Water looking like chocolate may be useful for washing and bathing purposes, not to mention culinary uses, but it is scarcely pleasant. Expedients for filtering the water within the reservoir have failed. It remains, therefore, that the water be filtered before it is pumped up to the main reservoir, and this can be effected by the following method: Construct a filtering basin at the head of the ravine in front of the Hospital, into which pump the water from the river; and construct a lake in the bottom lands into which the filtered water could flow and be stored. From this the main reservoir could be supplied. The pumps at the pump-house are abundantly sufficient for this additional work, and connections can be readily made. In this way an abundant supply of pure water could always be obtained.[7]

With Dr. John Snow's discovery of the transmission of cholera from a London water pump in 1849, municipal sanitary engineering was born. The first water filtration system in the United States was built in Poughkeepsie, New York, in 1872, and there typhoid deaths dropped as drinking water from the Hudson River was filtered through beds of sand. Just four years later the asylum trustees at Athens followed suit with a request for funds to build a filtering reservoir:

> It is imperatively necessary that the next work in grading should embrace the following distinct objects: first the filling up to a proper grade of the spaces designed for a kitchen-garden south of the male wards; and second, the excavation for, and construction of, a lake in the low land in front; and a filtering reservoir, so that at all times pure water can be pumped into the reservoir, from which the Hospital is supplied. At present the water is pumped directly from the Hocking River, which is often very muddy, and the water is then anything but desirable for laundry or other domestic purposes.[8]

The governor arranged for funding, and work on water purification began the next year, 1877: "The most important work of the summer has been looking to an increase of the water supply, and the means of purifying the water before its introduction into the house. This is being done by substituting larger supply pipes for the ones in use . . . and the construction of a storage reservoir in the bottom lands fronting the hospital. This work has been carried on as rapidly as possible, under the supervision of Mr. Haerlin, to whom we are indebted for the plan."[9] Haerlin designed a series of lakes and dams that he envisioned would supply the asylum with water and ice, provide beautiful scenery, and encourage boating activities: "The Legislature made an appropriation for building a storage reservoir and constructing filters, to purify the water before its introduction into the house. To this end, the bottom lands fronting the hospital, on being converted, under the supervision of Mr. Haerlin, into a beautiful lake which, when completed, will furnish storage capacity for at least four weeks supply of water . . . and the conversion of a miasmatic, disease-breeding bottom into a broad, healthful surface of living water, and a vast addition to the beauty and cheerfulness of the grounds and a source of ice supply."[10]

In 1878, Haerlin turned his attention to planting trees and creating a vegetable garden: "Under the direction of Mr. Haerlin, the transplanting of ornamental trees and shrubs to the space filled up by the grading of the previous season has taken place. . . . [T]he vegetable garden has been extended to a limited degree, and the whole raised to grade."[11] Assisting and eventually replacing Haerlin in the supervision of grading and planting was Athens townsman George Link.[12] Mr. Link provided the local leadership and supervision to execute Herman Haerlin's master plan for the asylum's landscape. The landscape reached its maturity in the twentieth century, as chronicled by the local newspaper in 1952:

> George Link . . . carried out the actual work of planning and his work took more than 30 years after 1873. More than 400 men did the grading and filling, leveling of hills and filling of ravines, planting scores of trees. The rounded slope in front of the main building is entirely artificial, as the refuse from the clay works and brick kilns where the brick[s] used [to build the asylum] were burned, was thrown into the place and graded. The lakes were built last and the earth removed was used to build the sloping drive on the river side. More than 18,000,000 bricks were made of clay from the surrounding hills. George Link surveyed and built the roads, graded the grounds and [saw to it] that the earth was slowly moved with manual labor and horse drawn vehicles. Now only one tree remains of the original timber, hundreds were shipped in and set out by George Link who staked out the groves. The result is conceded to be the most beautiful of any state institution in the Middle West.[13]

Mr. Link spent most of his career developing and tending the asylum's landscape. His obituary in 1903 is headlined "George Link, Landscape Gardener at Hospital for Thirty-two Years" and notes that "for the past 32 years he has had charge of the grounds of the state hospital, and as a result of his labor and skills, the institution has become noted for the beauty of its surroundings."[14] Born in Darmstadt, Germany, in 1932 and immigrating to America at the age of twenty-four, Link no doubt grew up appreciating the beauty of his town's Herrengarten, public grounds featuring statues and tombs of royalty, a military parade ground, trees, lawns, and fountains. After arriving in America, he married Catherine Eckle, an émigré from Prussia. They made their home in Athens, where they had five children, the first of whom was born in 1859. George and Catherine Link raised their children in their home directly opposite the entrance to the grounds of the Athens Lunatic Asylum. Paid by the asylum as a contractor rather than a staff wage earner, Link's title was grading foreman or simply grade boss.[15] Well paid for the time, George Link earned six hundred dollars for twelve months' employment, compared to assistant physicians, who earned seven hundred dollars per year.

Grading—smoothing out the extreme peaks and valleys of the site—was accomplished by means of teams of horses and mules dragging carts and large pans into which earth and rock had been shoveled by hand and drawn to areas needing filling. Blasting, achieved with hand grenades, was in some instances required to loosen the rock so that the land could be shaped. To accomplish this very labor-intensive process, at first Haerlin and later Link supervised a small army of hundreds of Athens townsmen and male patients, who worked alongside each other on this grading for the gardens and building waterworks, dams, lakes, and roads. The asylum's trustees, ever watchful of expenses, asked the legislature for money to complete this grading, which created the landforms on which gardens would be laid out. Large forces of men worked together at one time to take economic advantage of the supervisory experience of Haerlin and Link:

> We desire to call the especial attention [of] the Legislature
> to the unfinished condition for the grounds immediately
> surrounding the hospital, and the pressing necessity for
> a sufficient appropriation to complete the heavy grading.
> True economy demands that this be done at once, so that
> the work may be carried on to gradual completion by the
> ordinary labor of our own household, and that the skilled
> labor, at present a necessity, may be dispensed with. The
> longer this work is delayed by insufficient appropriations,
> the more expensive it becomes for the reason that
> it demands the constant supervision of a competent
> landscape gardener. This skilled labor may direct a large
> force of employees as readily as a small one, but is just as
> necessary with a small force as with a large one. In other
> words, the price of the skilled labor is the same whether
> the force of common laborers be large or small and the
> larger the force of common laborers the sooner can skilled
> labor be dispensed with.[16]

The labor contributed by patients at Athens and at most state asylums of the nineteenth century to alter landforms, create infrastructure, and maintain gardens saved the asylum money, kept patients occupied, and (according to their medical superintendents) made patients healthier. While the board of trustees dwelt upon cost savings of patient labor, asylum physicians discussed the benefits to patients in their reports to the Ohio Legislature. With few treatment modalities available in the nineteenth century, asylums relied on the labor of patients to fill their days, induce sleep at night, produce an appetite, and tone the muscles. In fact, the asylum superintendents considered the exercise and occupation afforded by the landscape the most curative aspect of patient care: "The condition of the patients is showing continued improvement [and we see] greater self-control and regard for property manifested by all. Abundance of outdoor exercise, and regular occupation of some kind, are the chief means by which this change has been effected."[17]

The superintendents began to set their male patients to work outdoors within a few years of the asylum's opening. Noted Dr. Rutter in 1876, "A large part of the out-of-door work has been done by patients, under the supervision of their attendants and others. They helped extensively in farming, in gardening, in grading, and to a lesser extent in the occupation of the shops. . . . [T]he only regret is that so many remain unoccupied, whom nothing can tempt to beneficial exertion. This is undoubtedly the great problem to be solved in the treatment of the insane—especially of the chronic insane—the development of industrial pursuits and the care of their health at the same time." Dr. Rutter continued, musing about the difficulty in convincing patients to work and the fine line between suggestion and compulsion: "'We did not come here to work' is so readily retorted when a patient is urged to some labor, and it is undoubtedly true, yet in many cases a few hours of moderate labor each day would be among the best of all remedial agencies. How to employ pressure and stop short of compulsion, for the good of the individual is not always easy of solution. The latter is not to be thought of."[18] A few years later, in 1881, Dr. Richardson noted the benefits of digging and shoveling fresh earth: "The chief problem is to furnish employment of a suitable kind, and in sufficient variety. One of the most healthful occupations is the digging and shoveling of fresh earth. A large force of men has been kept busy during the season for outdoor work in grading the grounds about the Asylum and [a] marked improvement [has been] made in the condition of the working men, both physically and mentally."[19]

The asylum's superintendents kept detailed records of patient work and its benefits. They noted the number of patients working outdoors each month, as well as the number of patients treated with chemical restraints such as sleeping medications and narcotics. Superintendent Richardson noted,

> There has been a daily average, for every working day in the year, of 137 patients who have been employed at some form of labor outside the wards. The work done has been in every case voluntary, though all proper inducements and arguments have been brought into use to encourage such a disposition. A variety of employments have been utilized: grading, gardening, fencing, painting and the various kinds of work in the different departments and with the mechanics about the institution. These [laborers] have been taken principally from the most disturbed wards, and the improvement has been plainly evident. . . . [I]f you can but induce a patient to apply himself methodically in some useful direction, you have gained strong gains with his disease. . . . [A]s a result fewer brawls and disturbances among patients have been noted. There has been a decrease in the number of complaints; a smaller amount of stimulants and medicines of all kinds has been found necessary. By reference to the tables [of annual statistics prepared by the superintendent] it will be seen that a daily average of less than five persons took any form of sleeping draught or narcotic medicine during the entire year. They have better appetites, and the record of noise and disturbance by night indicates of diminution in the amount. The patients are a better color and more rugged. Their muscles are firmer and they can endure more fatigue. They have more red blood. There is an absence of the sallow, cachectic and haggard countenance so common among this class.[20]

Superintendent Richardson elaborated on the role of patient labor in his 1883 report to the trustees and made the wildly progressive (for the times) recommendation that the state pay patients for their work, an idea that was acted upon by federal law nearly a century later.[21] Plainly, inducing patients to work was often difficult, and payment for their labor would make it easier to get them to do so by increasing their motivation.

> It has occurred to me in this connection as the result of what experience and opportunity for observation I have

had, that the benefits to be derived from the employment of the insane would be greatly increased by a moderate money remuneration. The chief object of such employment should always be the improvement of their condition, though to give proper zest the work done should be of practical utility. I believe a slight compensation only would increase their interest in their work, and, to a great extent, do away with that listless and dogged frame of mind in which they often pursue their occupation. It would give them a visible object for which they could labor, and tend to renew their interest in the future. It would also add to their feeling of responsibility while they are still under supervision, and thus better prepare them for the active work of life when discharged from the institution.[22]

Patients also worked in the asylum's fruit and vegetable gardens. The asylum needed vast quantities of food for the three meals a day prepared for seven hundred patients and upwards, as well as the staff, all of which was at first supplied by surrounding farmers and merchants. Superintendent Rutter established a kitchen garden, but two years later Superintendent Gundry found that the location was not suitable because floods regularly washed away the vegetables.

I can not too strongly urge the necessity of continuing the grading of this part of the premises, and to fill up with it the low place near the fence on the south designed for the kitchen garden. A part of the work has been done, sufficient to indicate the manner in which it is intended to finish the whole, but it ought to be pushed forward without delay, for dependence upon the bottom land in front for raising vegetables is a delusion. The soil is not adapted for a kitchen garden, and, moreover, it is liable to overflow and twice has the Hocking River carried off in summer within the past three years the product of the preceding summer's labor.[23]

Dr. Gundry went on to propose plans for more fruit orchards and a new location for the vegetable gardens to complement the success of the flower gardens and greenhouse built under the design and supervision of Mr. Haerlin.

Now the vegetables are raised in patches cultivated here and there, but it would be true economy to concentrate the work upon one spot. It is true it will take great labor to make the kitchen garden, but the results will, in my opinion, justify the toil and expenditure. I may add that during the past season we have enjoyed a goodly production of vegetables raised on the place, mostly by the labor of the patients. The orchard planted last fall is doing well, but a small proportion of the trees died, and will have to be replaced. Much more planting of fruit is required, and especially of small fruit, as soon as [a] place can be prepared for them. Our flower gardens and green-house have been very successfully cultivated, and have yielded pleasure to all sensible of the charms of nature. That part of the grounds already finished attests the skill and taste of the landscape gardener, Mr. Haerlin, and wins the admiration of all beholders.[24]

Ohio's governor provided funds for the kitchen garden, and the following year the asylum steward purchased fruit and vegetable plants on a vast scale, the planting of which was directed by Mr. Haerlin: "Under the direction of Mr. Haerlin the transplanting of ornamental trees and shrubs to the space filled up by the grading of the previous season has taken place. This required over . . . twenty thousand cubic yards of filling, covering an area of over seven (7) acres of surface."[25] The following fruit and vegetable plants were set out that year.

TABLE 5.1

Fruiting plants and vegetables planted in 1877

Fruits	*Seeds and vegetable plants*
86 apple trees	300 rhubarb plants
100 cherry trees	1,000 asparagus plants
100 plum trees	1,300 cabbage plants
25 peach trees	
450 currant vines	
754 grapevines	
100 gooseberry vines	
900 raspberry vines	
1,400 strawberry plants	

Source: Board of Trustees of the Athens Asylum for the Insane, 1885 annual report.

By 1883 the fruit and vegetable gardening operation was in full swing, with patients contributing most of the work to tend the gardens. In 1885, the asylum began reporting to the governor the results of the gardening effort. Wrote Dr. Richardson that year, "The garden has produced nearly all the vegetables, outside of potatoes, that we have used. Cabbage, tomatoes, corn, beans, peas, parsnips, beets, onions, pumpkins, turnips, asparagus etc. have been produced in quantities nearly sufficient to meet the wants of the institution, and by the labor of patients almost entirely."[26] Richardson also took the occasion to reaffirm the curative priority of outdoor work by patients, secondary to the practical matter of free labor. "Outdoor exercise in walking or working [are] all utilized for the one purpose—the financial return for the labor being held to be secondary to the beneficial effect upon the patient himself. Our ability to abolish mechanical restraint, to cut down seclusion to so low a figure, to almost abandon sleeping draughts, and to give so much individual liberty to so large a proportion is largely due to this feature of the treatment, and its importance cannot well be overstated."[27]

In 1885 for the first time the steward reported on the volume of fruits and vegetables produced from the asylum's gardens, as well as fruits canned. The huge amount of food produced and preserved by patients and staff made the asylum one of the larger market-garden producers in Ohio. Two thousand gallons of fruit were preserved in the asylum kitchens in 1886; two years later, production increased to six thousand gallons of preserved fruit.

In 1890 the asylum's entire fruit crop failed, likely because of late cold weather, and unbudgeted expenses were incurred to buy needed food. But three years later, the garden was especially successful and was expanded by the acquisition of four acres from a dairy farmer. Wrote the superintendent to Ohio's Governor William McKinley, "The results of the farming and gardening operations have been successful beyond our expectations. There had been but little purchased in the way of these products, except potatoes. We also have an abundance of canned tomatoes, cabbage, s[aue]rkraut, pickles and onions, all of which were raised, principally, by our patients' labor, stored for winter use."[28]

In addition to serving as a work site, asylum grounds at Athens and other asylums were used daily for exercise for female and male patients. Supervised outdoor group walks and unsupervised individual rambles constituted the centerpiece of treatment at the asylum at Athens. Dr. Richardson described his system:

TABLE 5.2
Garden production in 1886

Fresh produce	Amount	Canned fruit	Amount
Asparagus	544 bunches	Blackberries	57 gallons
Beans, Lima	57½ bushels	Cherries	745 gallons
Beans, string	144¾ bushels	Gooseberries	95 gallons
Beets	160 bushels	Grapes	56 gallons
Cabbage	11,000 heads	Peaches	81 gallons
Cauliflower	681 heads	Pears	112 gallons
Carrots	10 bushels	Plums	60 gallons
Celery	4,402 heads	Raspberries	227 gallons
Corn, green	1,900 heads	Strawberries	17 gallons
Cucumbers	3,026 dozen	Tomatoes	664 gallons
Gooseberries	14 bushels		
Lettuce	87 bushels	*Preserves, fruit butter, jellies, etc.*	*Amount*
Onion	121 bushels	Apple butter	262 gallons
Onions, young	92 dozen	Blackberry jam	12 gallons
Oyster plant	10 bushels	Currant jelly	14 Glasses
Parsnips	150 bushels	Grape butter	36 gallons
Peas	82 bushels	Peach butter	170 gallons
Potatoes	90 bushels	Raspberry jam	44 gallons
Pumpkins	1,070 bushels	Tomato preserves	5 gallons
Radishes	689 dozen	Various jellies	250 glasses
Rhubarb	685 pounds		
Spinach	65 bushels	*Other preserved foods*	*Amount*
Squashes	416 bushels	Cucumbers	36 gallons
Tomatoes	254 bushels	Cucumbers, salt	36 barrels
Turnips	163 bushels	Sauerkraut	21 barrels
		Spiced cherries	106 gallons
		Spiced currants	2 gallons
		Spiced peaches	18 gallons
		Spiced pears	29 gallons
		Tomato catsup	30 gallons

Source: Board of Trustees of the Athens Asylum for the Insane, 1886 annual report.

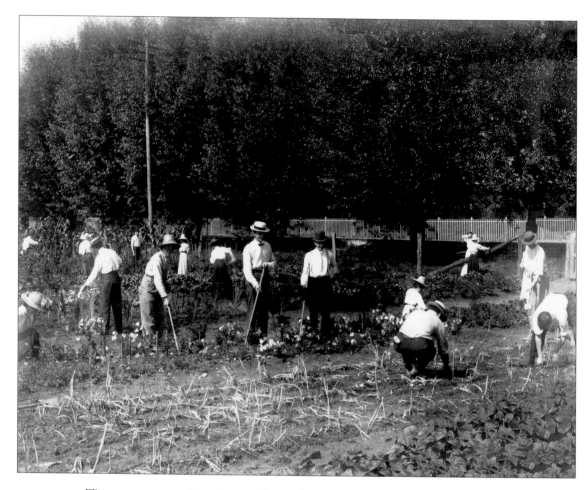

FIGURE 5.3 The asylum's gardens and orchards produced fruit and vegetables for nearly a century. This picture shows a similar, though smaller, operation in Athens, a school garden associated with Ohio University. Summer-Garden Students in the School Garden. *Souvenir Edition of the Ohio University Bulletin, Summer Term, 1914* (Athens: Ohio University, 1914), 102. *Courtesy of the Mahn Center for Archives and Special Collections, Ohio University Libraries.*

For the outside work extra attendants have been employed, who work with the patients and are held responsible for their care and safety. The use of the airing courts has been abandoned.[29] Morning and afternoon, whenever the weather has been suitable, the patients, when not at work either inside or outside, or those for whom no suitable work could be provided, have been taken out over the grounds under the charge of the attendants. They go in groups of [a] single ward, of . . . 25–40 patients each, and remain outside for hours at a time, either sitting under the shade of the trees or taking long walks over hills about the Asylum. But few remain indoors. . . . [T]he power of habit is not lost among the insane, and it can be made to work wonders almost in their management. For *every day of the year,* except Sunday, when the regular walks are omitted, including all kinds of weather, summer and winter, there had been a daily average of 235 patients taken out for exercise in this manner.[30]

Richardson wrote in 1883 of the usefulness of exercise in patient management: "The improvement of the patients in behavior while outdoors has improved. There has been much less destruction of shrubbery and bad language and improper conduct is seldom heard or seen. . . . [I]n the ward, too, there is improvement. The accidents are fewer, showing a better discipline among the patients. There is more contentment manifested, less of the constant requests to be sent home. This is more marked among the males than the females, as their habits . . . make them feel any restraint more severely. Improvement is also shown in the amount of seclusion required by day, and of sleeping draughts at night."[31]

According to moral treatment philosophy, gardens and pleasure grounds were essential to patient treatment and well-being. The Athens grounds included gardens, pleasure drives, walkways, open fields, and a series of lakes. The grounds provided a place for exercise, as well as beautiful views, both of which were considered curative. Superintendent Holden in 1879 asked for funds for landscape beautification to create better views: "Outside of the drive in front . . . the grounds make a very ragged appearance and present a deplorable contrast with the finished grounds in front of the female wards. They greatly mar the beauty and symmetry of the portion which has been completed. . . . [T]his improvement will transform a repulsive looking spot to a place of beauty, that our poor unfortunates who are necessarily confined in the wards may look out upon with pleasure and delight."[32] Superintendent Clarke complained that the unfinished front grounds presented an unattractive appearance both to the public and to patients: "The slope in front of the eastern division of the building . . . remains untouched and presents a forbidding appearance. It should be brought to harmonize with the gracefully finished lawn lying in front . . . as early as practicable, not only for the purpose of pleasing the public eye, which it is always well to do, but [also] . . . to present to the view of those who look out for relief a landscape marked by no violation of the laws of harmony. For surely no agency contributes more potently to the relief of a mind disturbed than strictly harmonious sensorial impressions."[33]

By the 1880s, ten years of work by patients and Athens townsmen under the direction of Herman Haerlin and George Link had resulted in a beautifully crafted landscape. Their efforts had created eight acres of lakes and views from the hospital windows of carefully landscaped grounds. The asylum's greenhouse staff and

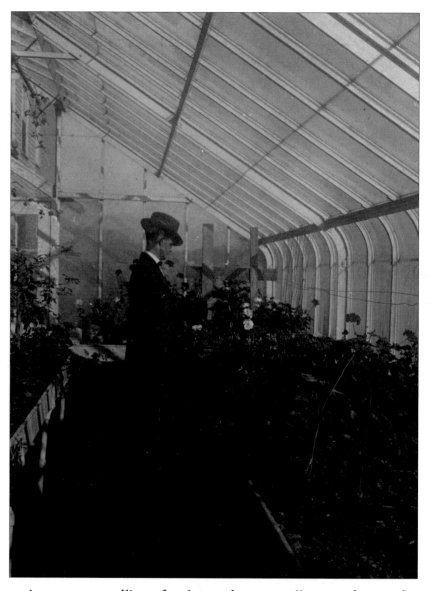

patients grew seedlings for the gardens as well as cut flowers for
the institution and the community. A florist was on the payroll
to see to floral and botanical ornaments for the wards and public
spaces, as well as cut flowers that were sometimes sent to important persons, such as the local newspaper editor.

The asylum landscape was a permeable boundary between the
institution and the community of Athens. Situated on its high bluff
above the river, the asylum was easily seen by the residents of Athens,
creating a visual connection. Both patients and townsmen mingled
as they labored on the grounds, and citizens and patients used the
grounds as parkland. In fact, the asylum grounds provided the only

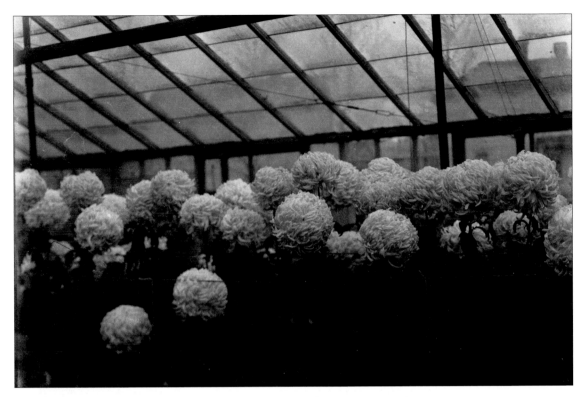

public park available to Athenians, who used it for picnics, ice-skating, walks, and other outings. An 1897 atlas of Athens County noted:

> Athens has no public gardens. Nature has done so much in the way of natural beauty that parks would seem to be a superfluity. . . . [T]he rugged hills . . . the fertile grass-covered lowland . . . the tortuous channel of the sometimes turbid Hocking, present a landscape as picturesque as can be found anywhere. The grounds of the Ohio Hospital, which comprise some two hundred acres, are highly cultivated and the fine natural park has been embellished with all the skill of the expert landscape gardener, and is surpassed by but few public gardens in any city. These grounds are always open to the public.[34]

FIGURE 5.5 Chrysanthemums growing in the asylum greenhouse. The asylum's florist provided arrangements for the wards and public administrative spaces and sent bouquets to important people in Athens such as the editor of the local newspaper. *Courtesy of the Mahn Center for Archives and Special Collections, Ohio University Libraries.*

The asylum once also opened its building to the people of Athens who needed shelter during a flood in 1907.

The landscape's permeability, however, sometimes presented security concerns. As the asylum neared completion, the trustees hired someone to guard the building. Patients working on outdoor projects sometimes took the opportunity to leave the asylum, or elope, in the terminology of the day. Male Patient 8, for example, admitted

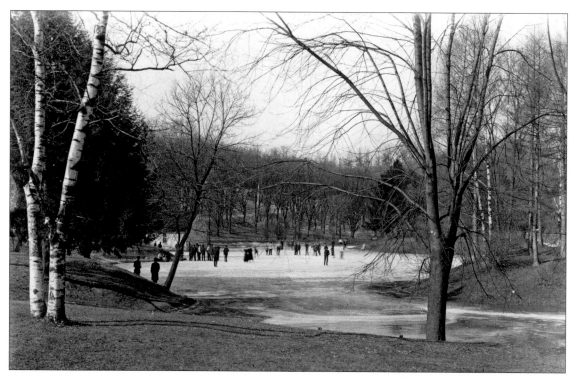

FIGURE 5.6 Skating pond on the asylum grounds. Residents of the village of Athens used the asylum's park-like setting year-round for recreation. *Courtesy of the Mahn Center for Archives and Special Collections, Ohio University Libraries.*

in January 1874 for attempting violence upon others, eloped that May. The entry in the asylum casebook notes that "he eloped while helping George Link fix the reservoir . . . nothing definite heard from him but said to be working on a farm in the South."[35]

Administrators had to be inventive to think of ways to keep patients from leaving and intruders from entering. In 1878, Dr. Clarke asked for money to plant a tall, prickly hedge around the perimeter of the grounds: "The hedge of Osage Orange should be planted without delay along the entire boundary. When matured, it will add very greatly to the beauty of the grounds, and will afford besides a fine protection against intruders, who now have such unlimited means of access, and a barrier in the way of those who are inclined to wander away from the Asylum."[36] The following year, Dr. Holden repeated the request for the protective hedge: "[I]t is highly necessary [that] we should have a hedge fence around the entire grounds. As it requires several years for its growth, the necessity of having it started immediately is obvious. Such a fence, when grown, will be almost a positive barrier against the escape of patients as well as a protection from intruders upon the grounds."[37] Succeeding superintendents may have been discouraged by the thought of the growing period, because neither a request nor an appropriation for a hedge fence appeared in subsequent annual reports.

Patient suicide was a constant concern for asylum physicians. At Athens, the medical superintendent had to balance the therapeutic benefits of the freedom to ramble unsupervised on the grounds with the risk of suicide. For this reason, only patients thought to be at no risk for self-harm were allowed this independence. Dr. Richardson presented his philosophy and its results in his report to the trustees: "The open door system begun by my predecessor, Dr. Rutter, has been continued and is being extended. The fact is recognized that the insane, in a large proportion of cases, are as favorably influenced by any exhibition of confidence reposed in them as the average sane person, and in each case the greatest individual liberty is given consistent with the safety of the patient and of those about him. It is really surprising how far this liberty can be safely extended when the attempt is carefully and thoroughly made. During the entire year not an incident of any kind has arisen from this cause."[38]

A year without a suicide in the asylum was unusual, however. During most years, a handful of patients were successful in completing suicides, and often the asylum grounds provided the site or the means. In 1883, for example, a female patient drowned in one of the lakes; circumstances were such that the county coroner was called upon to investigate the death, which was declared a suicide. "One suicide by drowning marks the one sad accident of the year. It was in the person of a female patient, an epileptic, who for many years had been allowed to take her daily walks about the grounds. Among that class of patients suicide is infrequent, and there was no thought of such a determination in her case. The Coroner was called upon, but exonerated all from any fault in the unfortunate occurrence."[39] Patients were separated by gender while outdoors; men and women patients were strictly forbidden to mingle. They were carefully supervised to prevent an "accident of an unfavorable kind that could be attributed to this grant of individual liberty," such as a pregnancy.[40]

Parklike settings and thriving agricultural operations were a hallmark of Kirkbride-style asylums in the nineteenth century. At Athens, the farming operations lasted into the 1970s. But this beautiful park landscape did not remain unchanged from Haerlin's design: it was drastically altered in 1968 when the Hocking River was rerouted as a flood-control measure, destroying the lakes, reservoir, and parkland that had served both the Athens community and the patients and staff of the asylum.[41]

SIX

CAREGIVERS

*"To Take Proper Care of the Insane Requires
Talents of a High Order"*

Chief Cook Elizabeth McCole walked through the empty kitchen on a Thursday night in 1887 checking the supplies she and her staff of five women would need for Friday morning. This was her thirteenth year of service at the asylum in Athens, having begun work there as a cook the year it opened. It was a big job, preparing three meals a day for nearly eight hundred patients, over a hundred staff, and the resident officers.[1] Tomorrow morning there would be buckwheat cakes, eggs, potatoes, and applesauce for patients; dinner at noon would be fish and boiled beef with bread and buttermilk; for supper, cornmeal mush with syrup and prunes, potatoes, meat stew, and bread and butter. The asylum's chief cook oversaw two kitchens: one that prepared meals for the officers and another for the patients and employees. The officers' table featured fine tableware such as silver butter dishes and water goblets.

Preparing three meals a day, providing clean laundry, and maintaining hygienic surroundings while also undertaking the psychiatric and medical care of eight hundred plus patients amid sometimes chaotic conditions such as suicide attempts, "noisy" patients, flickering gaslight, roads thick with mud, and problems with sewage was a considerable task. The moral treatment regimen at the asylum required the work of dozens of men and women attendants who provided direct patient care; specialized staff such as tinners, bakers, laundresses, cooks, engineers, firemen, upholsterers, gardeners, clerks, hostlers, seamstresses, and druggists; and a small professional staff of officers. Working together, they arranged for and supervised the outdoor airings and exercise, white-tableclothed dining rooms, fresh flowers, Sunday afternoon concerts, routine

TABLE SHOWING BILL OF FARE IN USE IN THE PATIENTS' DINING ROOMS.

[In addition to the bill of fare, such other vegetables and fruits as are not contained therein, as the seasons afford, are supplied.]

	Sunday.	Monday and Thursday.	Tuesday and Saturday.	Wednesday.	Friday.
Breakfast	Beefsteak	Mutton stew or sausage	Beef stew	Beefsteak	Mutton or pork.
	Gravy	Potatoes	Potatoes	Gravy	Buckwheat cakes.
	Potatoes	Hominy	Tomatoes	Potatoes	Eggs.
	Syrup	Syrup	Buckwheat cakes—syrup	Bread	Potatoes.
	Bread	Bread	Bread	Butter	Bread—butter.
	Butter	Butter	Butter	Apple sauce	Apple sauce.
	Apple sauce	Apple butter	Prunes	Rice	Hominy.
	Milk	Milk	Milk	Milk	Milk.
	Coffee	Coffee	Coffee	Coffee	Coffee.
Dinner	Beef, boiled and roast	Beef, boiled and roast	Mutton or pork; boiled or roast	Vegetable soup	Oysters or fish.
	Potatoes	Potatoes	Potatoes	Beef, boiled and roast	Beef, boiled and roast.
	Beans	Cabbage	Corn	Potatoes	Potatoes.
	Kraut	Turnips	Bread pudding	Beans	Beans.
	Bread	Bread	Kraut	Corn starch pudding	Cabbage.
	Butter	Butter	Bread	Bread	Bread.
	Pie	Corn bread	Butter	Butter	Butter.
	Milk	Milk	Milk	Milk	Milk.
	Coffee	Coffee	Coffee	Coffee	Coffee.
Supper	Beef stew	Beef stew	Meat stew	Beef stew	Meat stew.
	Potatoes	Potatoes	Potatoes	Potatoes	Potatoes.
	Bread	Bread	Bread	Bread	Bread.
	Butter	Butter	Butter	Butter	Butter.
	Apple sauce	Apple sauce	Syrup	Hominy	Cornmeal mush.
	Cornmeal mush	Oatmeal mush	Rice	Apple sauce	Prunes.
	Sugar cakes	Cheese	Apple sauce	Syrup	Syrup.
	Milk	Milk	Milk	Milk	Milk.
	Tea	Tea	Tea	Tea	Tea.

FIGURE 6.1 Weekly menu for the patients' dining room; the published menu was supplemented with fresh seasonal fruits and vegetables from the asylum's orchards and gardens. In 1891, the year of the publication of this bill of fare, the asylum kitchens served three meals a day to an average of 852 patients. Board of Trustees of the Athens Lunatic Asylum, 1891 annual report, 404. *Image provided by the State Library of Ohio.*

medical care, trips to town, and all the material needs for the entire asylum community.

The half dozen women staffing the asylum kitchens turned out three hefty meals a day for patients and staff. Meat and potatoes figured prominently at each meal, including breakfast. The published weekly patients' bill of fare for 1891 offered only prunes, applesauce, kraut, corn, cabbage, and turnips; fresh fruits and vegetables were limited to those produced by the asylum in its gardens and orchards.

By the mid-1880s the asylum's gardening operations, for which much of the labor was provided by patients, had begun to produce substantial quantities. Fresh string beans, radishes, spinach, tomatoes, squash, beets, cauliflower, celery, and other vegetables were harvested and served at the officers' table as well as to patients. Hundreds of gallons of fruit and vegetables were canned and preserved for use during the year: peach butter, raspberry jam, cherries, pears, plums, grapes, and gooseberries as well as tomatoes and pickles. The asylum's German-born tinner, Athens resident Frank Schloss, provided the kitchen staff with cans to preserve fruit. In 1886, the kitchen staff, with the help of patients, canned over a thousand gallons of cherries from the asylum's orchards. The farming operations also provided delicacies such as crates of strawberries for the officers' dining table as well as enough asparagus in the spring for staff and patients.

Before the new patient dining rooms opened in 1887, meals were prepared in the kitchen and taken to the wards. The new system of central dining rooms, one for male patients and one for female patients, allowed the kitchen staff to serve meals while they were fresh and hot. Each dining room had a serving room furnished with urns of hot tea and coffee and a large steam table for keeping food warm. When the food was ready, the kitchen sent a runner to signal the asylum's central exchange telephone operator to ring the wards and alert attendants to bring their patients. Wards One through Five, with quieter patients, ate in a dining room separate from the patients from wards Six through Nine, who were more disturbed (in the words of Superintendent Richardson). Plenty of staff was on hand to help; all attendants acted as waiters, and a physician was present in each dining room to make sure each patient was properly served and given enough time to eat. All in all, the staff felt that the large congregate dining rooms made for a more civilized dining experience for everyone—except the patients who were, using the psychiatric terms of the times, "unclean, paralytic and demented," meaning patients who could not move or who soiled themselves. These men and women, segregated in wards above the new dining rooms, took their meals in their rooms.

Some patients were permitted to walk freely about the asylum, which sometimes complicated things for the kitchen. Among the correspondence of superintendents kept in the asylum archives was a note from 1877 describing how William Buxton, an attendant helping out in the kitchen for the day, lost his temper with a patient who was going about soliciting from staff commitments of money and

FIGURE 6.2
Congregate dining room (for women), completed in 1887. Athens had the first asylum congregate dining rooms in the nation, an innovation from Superintendent A. B. Richardson. Family-style dining was thought to be therapeutic for patients, and because the time between cooking and serving was reduced, meals were fresher and hot. Before 1887, the food was ferried to the wards by a basement railroad system and lifts. *Courtesy of the Mahn Center for Archives and Special Collections, Ohio University Libraries.*

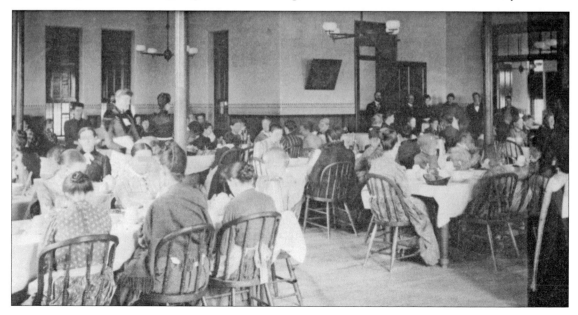

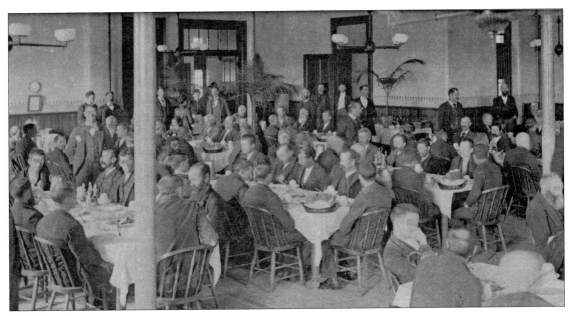

FIGURE 6.3
Congregate dining
room (for men),
completed in 1887.
Three meals a day
were served in the
dining room. *Courtesy
of the Mahn Center for
Archives and Special
Collections, Ohio
University Libraries.*

time to help build a church on the asylum grounds. Of course, the patient's plans for a church (complete with free transportation for patients in a horse-drawn bus driven by himself) were entirely his own. Buxton's supervisor wrote up the incident and sent it upstairs to Dr. Rutter, superintendent at the time: "Buxton in the kitchen got mad because _____ was taking subscription for church and flew off handle and ordered _____ out of the kitchen and tole him never to come back there again such damned business as that. _____ told him he [Buxton] could run the kitchen today and he would see further tomorrow after seeing his kind friend Dr. Rutter."[2]

Asylum staff supervised a sewing room in which women patients stitched aprons, bedding, dresses, shirts, skirts, tablecloths, towels, bonnets, and shrouds. In 1887, this sewing operation produced, among other items, 462 gingham aprons and 142 white ones, as well as over one thousand towels, 286 calico dresses, over three hundred skirts, and 513 pairs of drawers. The sewing room included at least one sewing machine, likely operated by a treadle as the asylum had no electricity until the mid-1890s. Among the list of purchases made by the asylum in 1887 were six dozen crochet needles, twenty-four dozen knitting needles, twenty-four pounds of yarn, and sixty-four pounds of knitting cotton, suggesting that patients and staff engaged in handwork such as knitting and crochet.

In addition to the kitchens and sewing room, women staffed the ironing room. Dora Barth, ironing room chief in 1887, supervised five women in the ironing room and three women responsible for washing and drying. This group of nine women had charge of all the laundry for nearly a thousand patients and staff. Equipped with

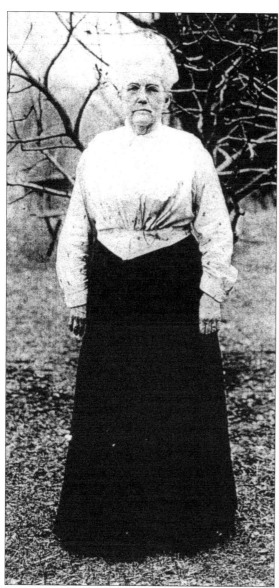

FIGURE 6.4 Postcard of Mrs. Sarah M. Clark, in charge of the asylum sewing room, 1879–1920. She was known by staff and patients as "Mother Clark." *Photograph courtesy of the Athens County Historical Society and Museum Photo Collection.*

newly refurbished washing machines and nine ironing boards, they laundered many hundreds of flannel and muslin drawers; as many dresses of calico, gingham, and lawn; shirts and waists; and the bath, table, and bed linens. In 1887, this staff was no doubt happy with one of Dr. Richardson's innovations designed to make the laundry work a little easier. He arranged for the trial use of a mangle, sent from New York City by the firm Hamilton E. Smith Esq. The mangle was a piece of machinery used for ironing by pulling down a heated flat surface on large items such as table linens. The mangle must have proved much easier than wringing and stretching by hand all the bed and table linens, as Dr. Richardson requested and received $550 from the governor to purchase the new automatic ironing machine.[3] Dr. Richardson also instituted a new staffing system for the forty men and forty women patients living above the dining rooms. He assigned night attendants who, by anticipating the needs and habits of their patients, reduced the number of soiled beds from twenty-five each night to two or three, creating that much less laundry for the ironing room chief to supervise.

FIGURE 6.5 (*opposite top*) Asylum night shift, 1893–94. Photograph taken on the steps of the front entrance. A system of night watch attendants was instituted by Superintendent A. B. Richardson to prevent patient suicides and reduce the soiling of bed linens. *Courtesy of the Mahn Center for Archives and Special Collections, Ohio University Libraries.*

FIGURE 6.6 (*opposite bottom*) Asylum day shift, 1893–94. Photograph taken on the steps of the front entrance. *Courtesy of the Mahn Center for Archives and Special Collections, Ohio University Libraries.*

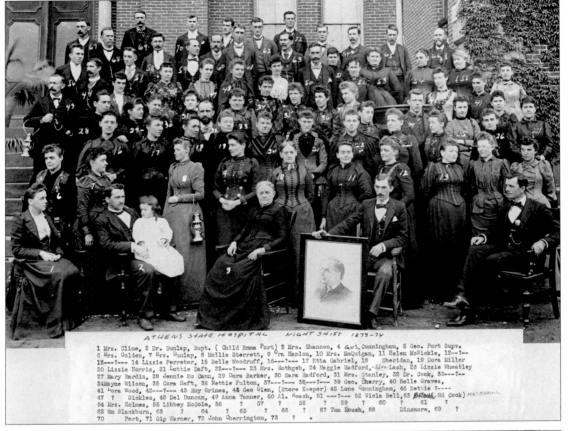

ATHENS STATE HOSPITAL   NIGHT SHIFT 1873-74

1 Mrs. Cline, 2 Dr. Dunlap, Supt. (Child Emma Port) 3 Mrs. Shannon, 4 Gus. Cunningham, 5 Geo. Port Supv.
6 Mrs. Golden, 7 Mrs. Dunlap, 8 Mollie Sterrett, 9 Dr Hanlon, 10 Mrs. McQuigan, 11 Helen McNickle, 12--?--
13---?--- 14 Lizzie Ferreter, 15 Belle Woodruff, 16---?--- 17 Etta Gabriel, 18   Sheridan, 19 Dora Miller
20 Lizzie Norris, 21 Lottie Daft, 22---?--- 23 Mrs. Rothgeb, 24 Maggie Radford,-24--Lash, 25 Lizzie Wheatley
27 Mary Rardin, 28 Jennie Mc Cann, 29 Dora Barker, 30 Sara Radford, 31 Mrs. Stanley, 32 Dr. Cook, 33---?---
34 Mayme Wilson, 35 Cora Heft, 36 Nettie Fulton, 37---?--- 38---?--- 39 Geo. Cherry, 40 Belle Graves,
41 Cora Wood, 42---?--- 43 Roy Grimes, 44 Geo Glen, (Store Keeper) 45 Lone Cunningham, 46 Nettie ?----
47 ?   Sickles, 48 Del Duncan, 49 Anna Tanner, 50 Al. Roach, 51 ---?--- 52 Viola Bell, 53 Brown Hd Cook) Mr? Brown
54 Mrs. Holmes, 55 Libbey McCole, 56   ?   57 ? 58   ?   59 ? 60 ? 61 ? ?
62 Wm Blackburn, 63   ?   64   ?   65 ? 66   ? 67 Tom Roush, 68   Dinsmore, 69   ?
70   Port, 71 Gip Warner, 72 John Cherrington, 73   ? .

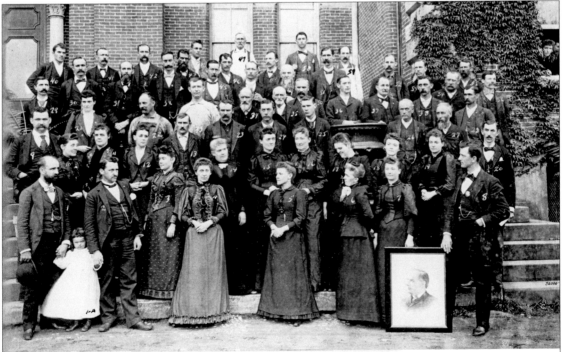

ATHENS STATE HOSPITAL   DAY SHIFT 1873-74

1 Dr. Cook, 2 Dr. Dunlap, 3 Mrs. Dunlap, 4 Mrs. Rothgieb, 5 Annie Lohi, 6 Abbie Hutchinson, 7 Eva Harrison, 8 Geo. Port
9 Dr. Wood, 10   Barker, 11 Mrs. Golden, 12 Mrs. Cline, 13   -?- 14 Mrs. Clark, 15   -?- 16 Emly Morrison
17 Etta Gabriel, 18 Jennie O'Neil, 19 Lottie Dick, 20 Gus Cunningham, 21 Lona Cunningham, 22 Dean Stickney, 23 Roy Brown
24   -?- 25   -?- 26 Hamilton Guiteau, 27   -?- 28   -?- 29 George Glen, 30 Roy Grimes, 31   Foster, 32 Al Roach
33 John Booth, 34   -?- 35 George Link, 36   -?- 37 George Barhart, 38 Tom Roush 39   -?- 40 Gip Warner
41   -?- 42   -?- 43 Ira Carscaden, 44   -?- 45   -?- 46 Wm. Rose, 47   -?- 48   -?- 49   -?-
50 Frank Schloss, 51 John Arhood, 52 John Lawrence, 53 Henry Dinsmore, 54   -?- 55   -?- 56   -?-
57   -?- 58   -?- 59   -?-

Dr. Agnes Johnson bent over the bed of the young woman who had been admitted that afternoon in need of restoration after childbirth. Leaving her baby and two small children with friends and relatives, she had made a hard journey of two hundred miles with her husband. Likely she agreed with a country physician in southeastern Ohio who wrote the superintendent of the need for small, well-run county hospitals where women such as this could recover from childbirth quickly and close to home. Puerperal mania was not uncommon among women in the asylum. In this instance, Dr. Johnson likely would have administered a sleeping draught of chloral hydrate to help her patient rest, left orders with the night attendant to encourage the patient to drink water should she awaken, and made a note to ask the kitchen to prepare a fortifying beef tea for her charge in the morning.[4]

Dr. Johnson shared the medical and psychiatric care of nearly four hundred women with one of the male assistant physicians. Dr. Richardson had hired her in 1881 to improve care for female patients at the asylum, a bold move praised around the state, from the governor's office to the Board of State Charities to the asylum's board of trustees. The first female asylum physician in the United States, Dr. Johnson was born in 1836 in McConnelsville in southeastern Ohio and received her medical education at the Women's Medical College in Philadelphia.[5] Part of the job of the asylum physician practicing moral treatment was to exert

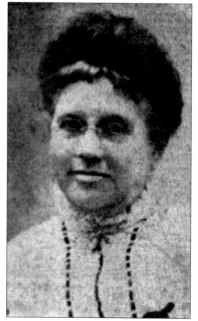

an elevating influence upon patients by their presence and interactions. At Dr. Thomas Kirkbride's Pennsylvania Hospital for the Insane, for example, the medical officers made daily rounds in the early years to visit patients considered most likely to benefit from their personal attention. By the 1880s, with 600–800 patients, the Athens asylum was too big for physicians to pay their patients daily visits. Dr. Johnson and her colleagues at Athens would have made an effort to do so with newly admitted patients, those who were critically ill, and patients who were mostly likely to benefit from their personal attention.

FIGURE 6.7 Dr. Agnes M. Johnson, assistant physician at the asylum, 1881–86, was the nation's first female asylum physician. She was hired by Superintendent A. B. Richardson to improve the care of female patients. *Photograph courtesy of Dr. Charles Cerney.*

1886 would have been a difficult year for Dr. Johnson, as her husband of thirty years had recently died. Years ago his health had failed, and he had to give up his work as a school superintendent, taking a quieter job as an insurance agent in Zanesville, Ohio. She had set up her medical office next to his branch office of the Connecticut Life Insurance Company to be nearby should he need her. Five years later they moved to Athens for her work at the asylum, where he died. Dr. Johnson was assisted in her work by a supervisoress and assistant supervisoress of the female attendants, as well as a night attendant. These women supervised the carrying out of the doctor's instructions and assisted in the care of very ill patients. In the event of the impending death of a patient, a physician or a supervisor would have kept a bedside watch. Another of Dr. Johnson's patients, an elderly woman suffering from dementia, had been brought to the asylum by the sheriff. Her family had waited until the last possible moment to take the step of asylum commitment, and when she arrived on the train, she lay near death, barely conscious with a bad cough and copious expectora. The casebook noted that her fever hovered around one hundred degrees and her pulse had increased from 98 to 120 beats per minute, and she had taken no nourishment. The staff must have recognized death approaching, because one of them sat with the patient until it came. Gripped by pneumonia, the patient died within a few hours of her arrival at the asylum. She was buried in a day or so in the cemetery on the hill, for her family could not make the long journey on roads six inches deep in mud to escort her body home for burial. In 1887, 67 of the asylum's patients died; about a third of them were buried on the asylum grounds.

Some of Dr. Johnson's patients recovered. One was admitted after having made recent attempts to destroy her life and that of her nine-month-old baby. Only twenty years old, unmarried, and living with her parents, who were of a religious nature, she was suffering from melancholia. Even though charities across the nation had begun to open homes for unwed mothers, in southeastern Ohio such women were usually stigmatized in their rural communities. At the asylum, she would have been treated with a plan of daily walks and perhaps some needlework with other patients and staff in the asylum's sewing room, to help her to regain her strength and enjoy a sense of community. Dr. Johnson, who left the employment of the asylum two years later to travel with friends in the United States and Cuba, likely never learned the results of her work with this patient, who within five years had recovered and married a farmer from her home county.

Steward Robert E. Hamblin sat at his oak desk on a spring evening in 1887 rechecking his accounting of purchases. The walls opposite Hamblin were lined with shelves that held twenty years' worth of purchasing accounts and payroll records. His office in the administrative section of the asylum was quiet, though he could hear the clatter of a wagon and horses. In his window the hills behind the asylum were black against the indigo evening sky, where a few pinpoints of stars were just appearing. The gas light sconces behind him sputtered, as they often did this time of year when the Hocking River rose with the spring freshet and covered the gas pipes that ran across the river, chilling the gas and restricting its flow. Soon, he hoped, the Athens Gas Light Company would agree to build and operate an electric plant for the asylum so the institution could be lighted by this clean and more reliable method. Or possibly he and Dr. Richardson would be able to convince the directors of the gaslight company to build the asylum its own new plant and supply electricity to the asylum. Either way, something had to be arranged soon. The nine-year contract he and Superintendent Richardson had negotiated with the company directors would come up for renewal in three years, and already the matter was an item for discussion at meetings of the board of trustees.

Robert Hamblin, steward of purchasing and payroll, and Dr. A. B. Richardson, medical superintendent, had a good working partnership. Born on a farm in nearby Hocking County, R. E. Hamblin had begun his career as an asylum steward at the age of twenty-five with Dr. Rutter in 1877; he and Dr. Rutter worked together again in 1880, and he was retained by the trustees when Dr. Richardson took charge.[6] The second oldest of farmer Enoch Everett Hamblin's four sons, Robert Hamblin managed the fiscal and payroll operations of the asylum with fairness and competence. He made purchasing decisions without much regard to politics, sometimes to the chagrin of businessmen, and he was known by vendors, staff, and politicians for honesty and fair dealings. Though he was a Democrat, Hamblin's forthright manner and business skills endeared him even to the Republicans who grumbled from time to time about his appointment as steward. His business skills were complemented by a fondness, and perhaps a political appreciation, for celebrations and public events. Christmas was marked with a Christmas tree and a turkey dinner for patients and staff, and the annual Fourth of July outdoor celebrations (open to the community) featured music, speakers, and plenty of food and were admired by the community.

The asylum steward was responsible for purchasing a stunning variety and volume of goods and services. Each year he purchased, among many other items, tons of cheese, hogsheads of New Orleans sugar, hundreds of pounds of candy, dozens of saltcellars, gallons of molasses, coffee, popcorn, salt, spices, steak pounders, woolen shirts, dozens of neck ties and handkerchiefs, birdbaths and birdseed, rat traps, spittoons, violins and violin strings, feathers, sawdust, straw, hay, lime, ice, honing razors, farm tools, blasting powder, padlocks, sewing machine supplies, dominoes, billiard balls, coffins, thousands of envelopes, and large volumes of whiskey, port, and brandy.[7] Drugs and medicines for the work of the physicians came from local businesses, and local African American hotelier Edward Berry sold barrels of oysters to the asylum. This year Hamblin had also purchased construction materials for new pigpens and a cattle shed: seventeen thousand board feet of oak, one thousand feet of oak flooring, and over nine hundred feet of poplar; two barrels of cement; and fifteen wooden doors. This amounted to a total investment of almost $900, but by raising its own beef and pork the trustees and officers believed the asylum would save money. The steward had also spent $1,200 for ten thousand pounds of South Carolina smoked ham; that time- and space-intensive commodity would be one he would continue to purchase rather than take in-house.

The asylum was a market for Athens farmers, from whom the asylum steward purchased great quantities of food year round. Some, especially the dairy and poultry farmers, were large operations, and the steward also purchased small quantities, such as five gallons of apple butter and a few dozen eggs. Most of the farmers with whom the steward did business were men, but a few Athens women were suppliers. A Mrs. William Coates supplied her buttermilk and cream a few gallons at a time, and Mrs. Mary Rice sold hay from her farm. The steward was busy year-round every year procuring farm produce for the asylum kitchens; in the summer it was fresh fruits and vegetables such as potatoes, plums, blackberries, rhubarb, melons, peaches, peppers, quinces, and sweet potatoes; in autumn the steward shopped for turkeys, apples, cider, dried apples, geese, and hogs; even in the winter he was busy purchasing dressed turkeys and a Christmas tree.[8] After the asylum gardens and orchards became productive, the steward continued to supplement the asylum harvests with local farm produce. In 1887, for example, the steward purchased thirty-five hundred pounds of rhubarb for the asylum kitchens to use for stewing and pie-making.

In addition to food, the steward purchased from local suppliers manure for the summer garden (eighty-seven wagon loads of it in 1887). Equipment to keep the asylum running was on the shopping list of the steward each year. In the late 1880s, asylum engineer James Bruner ran the heating and water works for the institution with the help of two assistant engineers, four firemen, and coal wheeler Lemuel Oxley; Bruner and his team were in constant need of new hardware such as valves and steam traps for repairs and extensions. Furniture was always needed, as it took heavy wear from the eight hundred–plus patients. In 1887, even with $125,600 in anticipated receipts from the State of Ohio, there would not be enough for the two hundred wooden beds needed to replace worn and dilapidated ones. A few patients were sleeping on mattresses on the floor that year, and the steward would have only enough funds to buy a few beds to get patients off the floor. The steward was also constantly busy making arrangements for the construction of improvements and making repairs. In 1887, he supervised the construction of two new fire escapes for the infirmary manufactured by the Motherwell Iron Works of Logan, Ohio. In addition, each month every year the steward prepared the payroll and managed the bid-taking process for the asylum's contracts for coal, gas, meat, and milk.

Lucinda Pickett sat writing at a small table in Female Ward 7 in 1874, taking a few moments there before leaving her patients for the night. It had been a long day, though since the weather had been fine she had been able to take a few of her patients for a walk outdoors. Helping them dress in the morning, bringing them their meals, and organizing their afternoon walk had absorbed most of her attention all day long. She thought she would relax for a moment and write a letter to her mother before having her own supper and then retiring for the night to the dormitory room she shared with another attendant at the back of the asylum. Her fountain pen filled with purple ink moved quickly across the lined note paper.

Lunatic Asylum April 23, 1874

My verry Dear Mother
I must tell you something about how I am getting along. My health is good but I get awful tired being on my feet so much. I am in No. 7 the worst ward in the House

we have thirty five Patients. I have just finished combing their Heads you better believe I had a time getting them combed I had to fight some of them to get them to sit still. I believed in Moral Suasion until I came here but it dont do here you have to be Prompt to get along with the Patients. I expect you would like to know something about how I arranged my Business.

I rented my House to Dave Maryburgh for one year the rent to be applied on the Property subject to my order. Annie is Living at Ann Ballards she is getting along verry well she was over this week and Brought Mrs. Ballards Little Girl with her. I had a Letter from Minnie the other Day she says she is not one bit home sick she wrote a real funny Letter. She is Living at Mr. Will Craigs near Nelsonville they are good Pious People they are going to send her to school this summer. They have two Little Children.

You don't know what a week of trials it was to me the week I came down here when I Packed up my goods and separated My Family. One of my Children went one way and the other the other way to Live with strangers. Minnie said she wanted to go [with] the man and his wife. . . . Poor child it nearly killed me to see her go but I thought it was for the best, even now while I am writing I have to shed Tears. This is what keeps my heart from Breaking Oh what a relief to go away by yourself and take a good Cry when you are in trouble but enough of this. The Good Lord will deal justly with us and I feel like Bowing in humble submission.

Well you may tell all the folks to write to me I can't write to Amanda for I don't know where to write I hope none of them will wait for me to write. My wages here will be Fifteen Dollars Per Month. I can save the most of that it Don't cost me any thing to Live here only Clothes. I can do better here than I could sewing. And I get Plenty of sleep and Plenty to eat and that is good enough for any body.

I hope you will look over all Mistakes there is so much confusion here I cant write worth a cent.

Let me hear from you soon
Your Child
L. Pickett[9]

Lucinda had sent her children to live with other families out of necessity. With no husband or other family to help, and money and work scarce, she had been successful in obtaining a position as an attendant at the asylum when it opened. Required to live on the site and desperate to provide for her small family, she had obtained a small monthly income to send to her daughters, and she could avoid the charity of the county home, or the "poorhouse." Lucinda was willing to work hard and had heard of moral treatment philosophy. But with no training except what she received at home, she as well as other employees found attending to patients with mental illness difficult and would not stay long. Public asylums across America had trouble from their inception with retaining attendants because of the difficulty of the work. At the Manhattan State Hospital for the Insane on Ward's Island, in 1875, only two attendants had worked there for more than twelve months. Worcester Hospital, at the end of the nineteenth century, saw turnover of its attendants of at least twice per year. Their curative work of providing useful occupation and an elevating environment was compromised by their responsibilities to bathe and dress patients, clean the wards, and make and change beds. They dealt with disorganization and constant threats of disruption, prompting many to leave and others to respond with violence toward patients with difficult behaviors.[10]

By June, Lucinda Pickett had married a sixty-year-old widower, George Connett, who provided a comfortable life for Lucinda and her daughters. Two years later she would write to her mother that "Mr. Connett is the best man I ever saw I think; he is so kind and tender I don't want for any thing that can be Bought for money."[11] Thirteen years after Lucinda had left her job as an attendant, turnover among attendants at Athens had dropped; the asylum officers had learned that the practice of hiring attendants with no training and little experience led in some instances to abuse of patients and that supervised time on the job was valuable training. Wrote Dr. Richardson in his 1887 annual report,

> The changes among the force of employees during the year have been unusually infrequent. With 132 on the pay-rolls of the institutions there were but 21 changes from all causes. The lapse of time has enabled us to establish a permanency and secure an experience that is highly gratifying to all who can appreciate the value of these features in the care of the insane. It requires from six months to one year for an attendant to get such a knowledge of his duties as will enable him to render efficient service. With 59 day and night attendants there

were but nine changes . . . [and] 35 of the 59 attendants have been in service for three years or more.[12]

With four professional staff (the superintendent and three assistant physicians) looking after 780 patients by 1887, the fifty-six attendants on staff were primary caregivers. Dr. Richardson began building a rationale for a professional cadre of trained asylum attendants:

> I take great pleasure in commending the entire corps
> of employees for the interest they have shown in the
> discharge of their duties. It is difficult to conceive a more
> responsible work than that in which they are engaged. The
> insane are not only helpless as far as their own interests
> are concerned, but have added, by their disease, such
> propensities as render them sources of irritation to those in
> charge of them. To take proper care of the insane requires
> talents of a high order. Attendants should be persons
> of more than ordinary intelligence, and should have an
> absolute command of their temper. The combination of
> qualities required is not often found, and the selection of
> attendants should therefore be most carefully made, and
> every legitimate inducement should be held out to suitable
> persons to continue permanently in the work. It is a
> specialty, and should really take rank as a profession.[13]

Attendants worked with patients with a great variety of temperaments and behaviors and had to be on the watch for patient self-harm. Usually one or more patients succeeded in committing suicide each year, often by drowning in the new lakes or walking in front of a train on the nearby tracks. In the early twentieth century, American asylum attendants began to receive formal training. Attendants at the Texas State Lunatic Asylum were instructed to be watchful for the various means by which patients might seek to end their lives:

> Drowning in bathtubs; cutting wrists and neck with eye
> glasses . . . and window panes; strangulation by . . . pajamas,
> . . . towels and bed clothes; standing in high places such as
> . . . window sills, beds and falling on head; use of scissors,
> occupational tools, knives, forks, spoons etc; tipping a chair
> over backwards . . . drinking cleaning solutions; starvation;
> picking the body to obtain infection; knocking head
> against the wall; running head first through panes of glass;
> jumping off walls; and falling on head down the stairs.[14]

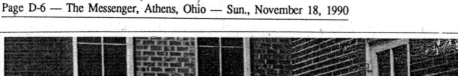

FIGURE 6.8 Dr. Alonzo B. Richardson; photograph taken while he was superintendent of St. Elizabeths Hospital, Washington, D.C. *Courtesy National Archives, photo no. 418-DP-49.*

Dr. Richardson in his 1887 report wrote of the gratifying lack of suicides ("fatal accidents") that year but noted the success of one man in completing a chilling act of self-mutilation. "The results of the year's work have been as favorable as could have been anticipated. We have had no fatal accidents among the patients, and the affairs of the Institution have moved along in a quiet way with but little to call for comment. There have been the usual and unavoidable minor casualties, among them being an occasional fracture of a bone, and in one strange but interesting case, the self-mutilation of his body by a male patient, by the cutting off of his right hand."[15]

FIGURE 6.9 Asylum nurses helping prepare Thanksgiving dinner, 1913. *Photo courtesy of the* Athens (OH) Messenger.

Twelve years later as superintendent at Ohio's Massillon State Hospital, Richardson established plans for a nursing school there. By 1911, the Athens asylum had affiliated with it a training school for nurses with a three-year curriculum.[16]

Mr. James C. Bowers, dairy farmer, packed up his tools and headed out the back door of the asylum kitchens. He had stopped that day in 1887 to deliver milk, install several items from his

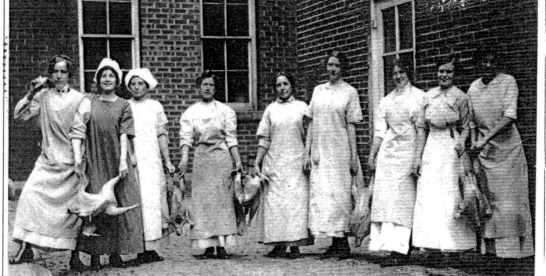

blacksmith shop, and make a few repairs. This year was his tenth of doing business with the asylum, the main portion of which was his annual milk contract. His first annual contract, for twelve cents per gallon of milk, earned him $2,744 for providing over 22,000 gallons of milk. Since then his price had increased by just a penny, to thirteen cents per gallon, but he now supplied more than double the volume of milk he had sold for that first contract in 1877.[17] Born in 1842 on a farm in Ohio, when he was twenty Bowers married Catherine Runnion. He enlisted in the Ohio Infantry Fifty-Second Regiment and served until the end of the Civil War.[18] Their first child, daughter Erva, was born in 1863 while Bowers was away fighting. He returned in 1865, and the next year the first of five sons was born to the couple. When their oldest son, Newton, turned twenty-one, the youngest—twins Herbert and Herman—were fourteen. With his wife and children, Mr. Bowers ran the large dairy operation, which grew with the number of patients at the asylum. He often remained after his milk delivery to repair small items such as the kitchen's coffee roaster and install items made in his blacksmith shop. In 1887, he and his sons had made and installed several four-foot-long iron bolts and two rods for the asylum slop cart, which contained scraps of uneaten food, or swill, for the asylum's piggery.

Mrs. Julia D. Richardson, matron of the asylum and wife of Superintendent Alonzo B. Richardson, paused on the landing as she descended the stairs from the third floor of the women's wards on her way to the amusement hall. She had been checking to see that the windows in the rooms of female patients were closed against the cool of the April evening. That afternoon she had the windows opened so that the sun-warmed fresh air could circulate among the bedridden women in the ward. This evening she was feeling a little queasy and looked forward to a light supper with her husband and the other officers—a bit of food would stave off the nausea of early pregnancy, for Mrs. Richardson was a few months pregnant with her fourth child.

State asylums in the nineteenth century hired a matron to oversee the nonmedical care of female patients, and she was usually the wife of the superintendent. Dr. Richardson had married well, for his wife apparently had the energy, temperament, and skills to manage her work and complement his role as a superintendent. Following his first institutional work as a West Virginia school principal and then physician for a county jail, Dr.

Richardson began his asylum work at Athens and then moved on to Columbus, Ohio, before ending his career at the prestigious St. Elizabeths Hospital for the Insane in Washington, D.C. Julia Richardson was assisted in her work by assistant matron Hattie Golden. Mrs. Golden had begun employment at the asylum in 1885 as housekeeper. Her position was renamed assistant matron and her duties adjusted so that she directly assisted the matron. They would have worked together to plan social occasions such as the asylum's Sunday afternoon concerts, which were open to the public. The concerts were not as elaborate as those at Kirkbride's hospital in Philadelphia, which featured nightly entertainments such as magic lantern shows, speakers, concerts, plays, and exhibitions of singing canary birds.[19] However, the second floor amusement hall, a 2,600-square-foot frescoed room with a 28-foot-high ceiling, could be arranged to accommodate a large audience that often included townspeople from Athens.

The two worked closely with supervisoress Dora Barker, who had direct charge of all the female attendants. All three women received wages. Mrs. Richardson's annual wage as an officer was $400; Mrs. Golden received $300, and Miss Barker $240. By way

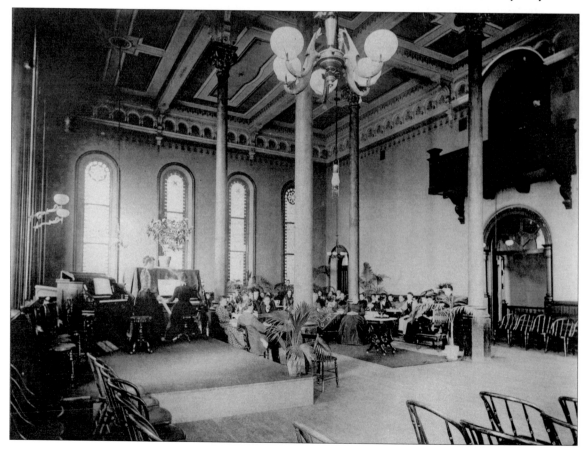

of contrast, the superintendent was paid $1,200 per year, his assistant physicians $700, and steward Robert Hamblin $800.[20]

Mrs. Richardson would have had daily opportunities to look through the asylum's glass windows across the river to the town of Athens, which had grown since she was born there in 1855. From the great asylum building on the ridge above the river she would have been able to see down to Court Street, by 1887 lined with merchants, hotels, and the handful of buildings that constituted Ohio University. She had met Dr. Richardson in 1872 when she was seventeen and he was twenty and about to graduate from the university and take up a position as principal of a school across the Ohio River in Ravenswood, West Virginia. For four years he courted Julia, daughter of Mr. James Wesley Harris of Athens, while he studied medicine under Dr. D. B. Cotton of Portsmouth, Ohio, and then at Bellevue Hospital Medical College in New York City. When he graduated from Bellevue, he returned home to Ohio, married Julia, and worked for one year as an assistant physician at the asylum at Athens, where their first child, William, was born. The staff was reorganized after only one year when Richard Bishop, a Democrat, was elected governor of Ohio, and Dr. Richardson moved with Julia and William to Portsmouth on the Ohio River, where he joined Dr. Cotton's practice and served as physician for the city jail. Dr. Rutter tried to get Dr. Richardson to return to Athens the next year as assistant physician, but Richardson had had enough of moving around and decided to settle in Cincinnati, where he built a large and comfortable home for his growing family, anticipating living there for many years. But before the house was completed, he was asked in 1880 by the governor to serve as the superintendent at Athens, Dr. Rutter having been called to superintend the asylum at Columbus. The opportunity was too good to pass up, so Dr. Richardson and Julia moved back to Athens, their family having grown by one with the birth of Mary Bertha. Soon after their arrival in Athens, their daughter Edith was born, and Julia Richardson as a young woman of twenty-four and mother of three took up her duties as asylum matron. Her career as an asylum matron took her from the rural isolation of Athens, Ohio, to the state capitol of Columbus and finally to Washington, D.C., as the matron of St. Elizabeths Government Hospital for the Insane. Her work in Athens overseeing the living conditions of four hundred female patients and planning Sunday afternoon musical concerts gave her the experience she needed for Washington, with twice the number of patients and a far more glittering social community.

Among the many duties of a nineteenth-century asylum superintendent was managing correspondence with families making inquiries and requests. At Athens, a relative of a patient wrote asking the superintendent to convey the news of the death of a patient's mother. The patient was a thirty-nine-year-old man admitted to the asylum in 1878 because of "incoherency with marked paroxysm of laughter, and attempts at violence."[21] The man had been in and out of asylums at Dayton and Cincinnati for the previous ten years, and his family feared the effect of the news. The relative wrote to the superintendent,

> Dear Sir
>
> I write through you to communicate the sad news of the Death of _____'s Mother she died last Friday Sept. 3 at 4 o'clock in the afternoon. I would have written to _____ concerning the illness of his mother but was fearful of the result. I take this method of communicating to him the news. . . . I hope that you will tell him in a way that it will not be injurious. You can tell him that she died Happy and wants him to meet her in Heaven. Please to answer and let me know how he receives it if he can Bear it. I will write to Him & give the particulars of her death and burial.[22]

The family of a thirty-three-year-old man hospitalized at Athens in 1876 because of attempts of violence against others wrote the superintendent with a change of address. The superintendent had written to the family requesting clothing for the patient, but because of a change of address, the shipment of clothing was delayed. The family wrote to explain and ask for news of their family member: "Sir I . . . would like for you to change the address. . . . That is what caused the Delay. Please let me know when you receive this and also state how his health and mind is." Enclosed with the letter was a small photograph of a woman in a chair, labeled "From your Mother."[23] Families wrote letters to asylum physicians asking about the advisability of visiting a patient. A young man wrote to Dr. Kelly, an assistant physician at the asylum, about visiting his brother on his way to college. "Dear Sir, It is now but a few days before I must return to my college duties at Marietta and myself and cousin would like to stop on our way back and see _____ if possible.

Late reports from you would lead us to think that this will be possible. Now I should like to know if we can do this without doing the patient any harm. We shall probably go by Athens the 6th of Sept. and if you will inform me as to this above you will oblige (me)."[24]

Much correspondence to and from families was in regard to patients' clothing. Patients' family or friends were required to provide clothing, although the state provided clothing for those with no resources. A probate judge wrote to Superintendent Holden in 1880 about the clothes accompanying a patient sent to the asylum from Chillicothe, Ohio: "Dear Sir—I sent you a patient today—He has all the outside clothing necessary—but not under clothing. His residence is fifteen miles away—I will see that the underclothes are brought in and sent down—I did not think best to have some bought when he has plenty at home."[25] Superintendent Holden wrote an acknowledgment of receipt of clothing for the patient: "2 shirts, 2 pr. Cotton socks, under Clothing, 2 Handkerchiefs, 1 felt Hat, 1 necktie."[26]

Superintendents wrote to families advising them about the condition of their family members, especially when they were ill. Superintendent Henly Rutter wrote to a family about a seventy-four-year-old patient, a Freemason who had become paralyzed on one side and suffered memory loss and hallucinations. Described by medical witness Dr. A. B. Richardson as a "rather free liver," he had suffered business losses, and after two years of caring for him his daughters had committed him. His granddaughter wrote to Dr. Rutter, "Your letter was received and we are very sorry to hear that Grand pa is failing so fast. Ma was away when your letter came to hand and I do not know when she will return. His other daughter . . . is anxious to hear from him. So pleas address her to this place and when Ma returns we will see what can be done for him."[27]

By the mid-nineteenth century, psychiatry had become a medical specialty in America. The forerunner of the American Psychiatric Association, formed in 1844 as the Association of Medical Superintendents of American Institutions for the Insane, established asylum superintendents at the forefront of the new specialty that had arisen to direct and staff the public asylums. It was in many ways an attractive bargain for asylum physicians: in exchange for taking charge of mentally ill persons, who were often troublesome members of their communities, asylum physicians would have well-paid, secure jobs and the opportunity to experiment with moral treatment, a novel way to heal persons with mental illness in new state-of-the-art public institutions.[28] But as the number of asylum patients grew, superintendents' jobs became administrative and managerial rather than curative. Formal and rigid procedures and processes replaced the flexibility superintendents and their assistant physicians needed to provide moral treatment by adjusting the environment of individual patients.

By the late nineteenth century, new models of care—the cottage plan of asylum architecture and research-based hospitals—had come to the forefront, bringing a close to moral treatment at state asylums across America, including at Athens. Moral treatment was literally grounded in bricks, mortar, and landscape: psychiatry had pinned its hopes for treatment and cure of mental illness on the asylum building itself and its extensive grounds. What followed both nationally and at Athens was a half century of custodial care in these very large and extensive buildings and grounds, then a transition to a variety of services and medications delivered in settings as varied as patients' homes and places of work, group homes, community art studios, the offices of primary care physicians, community health centers, community mental health centers, small inpatient mental hospitals, respite care centers, and institutions such as schools, prisons, and general hospitals.

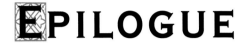PILOGUE

The End of Moral Treatment

In the summer of 1894, asylum superintendents from all over America convened for their fiftieth annual meeting. They gathered in Philadelphia, where half a century earlier the American moral treatment experiment in psychiatry had begun with Dr. Thomas Kirkbride's work at the Pennsylvania State Hospital. At this meeting of the American Medico-Psychological Association (formerly known as the Society of the Medical Superintendents of the Insane), neurologist Dr. S. Weir Mitchell delivered a point-by-point critique of America's asylums and their medical superintendents, many of whom were in his audience. Dr. Mitchell, who had founded the American Neurological Association in 1875 and was its first president, had been invited to give the keynote address and in preparing his remarks had surveyed neurologists across the nation about the "management of the insane in America," its faults, and suggestions for changes.[1] From the political boards that controlled asylum appointments, to a lack of scientific reports or case studies among the lengthy farm production and purchasing annual reports, attendants with no training, and the "superstition" of the curative nature of moral treatment and its architecture, to the role of the asylum superintendent as business manager and farmer, Mitchell excoriated American asylums, calling them boardinghouses with bad food and locked doors. In his address he described how patients in public asylums "sit in rows, too dull to know despair, watched by attendants; silent, grewsome [*sic*] machines which eat and sleep, and sleep and eat."

What did Dr. Mitchell propose? A new architecture of asylums, the cottage plan, which would segregate patients according to their ability to pay for their treatment. It should be

near to a city, its grounds fenced in not by walls, but by
railings vine covered and hidden by trees and shrubs . . . and
include some forest and wide, cheerful gardens . . . [with]
farm and vegetable garden . . . [with] a hospital . . . made
up of grouped cottages, each with its family or ten or twelve
or less, in each a head nurse and attendants. . . . [A]part
stand smaller [individual] homes for those able to pay
more. At a distance, hidden by trees, is the administration
building, vine clad . . . and flanked by the wards for those
who can pay little or nothing . . . with library, reading
rooms, billiard and amusement rooms . . . tennis . . . work
shops . . . school rooms.

These new cottage plan asylums would be supervised by physicians
who conducted laboratory research on the treatment of mental illness and staffed by cadres of trained psychiatric nurses.

Although moral treatment had achieved a degree of success in
treating mental illness, American academic psychiatry had shifted its
focus from asylum-based medicine to its twentieth-century inception as a research-based modern medical specialty.[2] Asylum medical
superintendents no longer enjoyed the status they had attained during the moral treatment era; asylum medicine had become a medical backwater compared to the emerging medical field aligned with
science and technology.[3] Whereas practitioners of moral treatment
asylum medicine were grounded in the work of reform-minded
Quakers (Kirkbride, for example, was a Quaker as well as a physician
and led his patients in Sunday evening Bible reading),[4] the newly
emerging psychiatry was founded on the empiricism of science.

Dr. Mitchell, in castigating asylum medicine, had said little
that asylum physicians themselves had not already said in their
reports to their trustees. American asylum superintendents had
since the 1880s described in their annual reports the difficulty of
maintaining moral treatment. They were overwhelmed and discouraged by crowded conditions, the great numbers of patients,
and the seemingly incurable nature of the elderly with dementia and patients with chronic mental illness. Even in Ohio, said
to possess one of the best systems of state asylums in the nation,
moral treatment had become difficult to practice by the late 1880s.[5]
The Athens asylum's Superintendent A. B. Richardson in 1889
noted that because he was responsible for so many patients it was
no longer possible for one medical superintendent with a handful
of assistant physicians to supervise moral treatment properly. At

Hilltop asylum in Columbus, Ohio, superintendents were unable to meet with their patients daily.[6] Citing a growing recognition of the importance of a trained cadre of supporting staff in a hospital for persons with mental illness, just before Richardson left Athens in 1889 he recommended establishing a psychiatric nursing school for the asylum, developing the work of asylum attendants as a psychiatric specialty, and building a research lab and a hospital wing devoted to care for patients who might be curable.

The new cottage plan of asylum architecture had actually been part of a proposal as far back as the 1850s by Dr. John Galt, superintendent of the Eastern Lunatic Asylum at Williamsburg, Virginia, for decentralized community-based care. This model in turn harked back a thousand years to the town of Gheel in Belgium, a religious shrine where persons with mental illness were sent for cure; by the nineteenth century, Gheel had developed a system of board and care for persons with mental illness with families in the town.[7] Galt's mid-nineteenth-century suggestions for decentralized care were criticized and then ignored, but the concept of decentralization of care for persons with mental illness, not to reach its zenith for another century with the deinstitutionalization of state mental hospitals, was incorporated into existing Kirkbride-style asylums around the nation with the addition of cottage-style architecture.[8] In Toledo, the entire new State Hospital, opened in 1883, was designed and built according to the new cottage plan.[9]

A Half Century of Custodial Care

What began in the nineteenth century as a quasi-religious reform movement grounded in principles of well-being that have been around for over two thousand years became during the first half of the twentieth century a public health near-disaster in America's state asylums. At Athens as across the nation, the second half of the twentieth century was spent digging out from the situation.

The asylum at Athens along with public asylums nationwide transitioned from moral treatment to custodial care. In Athens in 1903, three cottages (named O, R, and M) were built for patients. Treatment focused on keeping patients safe and occupied with working on the grounds, in the kitchens, and in the sewing room. The farm operations thrived. Patients and staff enjoyed clean drinking water, thanks to funds for the legislature for enlarging the lakes and installing filters. Wastewater treatment was another matter: the Village of Athens complained to the State Board of Health about the asylum's practice of emptying its sewage into the Hocking River, in which it flowed downstream and combined with wastewater from the county courthouse, polluting wells and causing bad odors. The State Board of Health eventually used Athens as a model for the investigation of a solution that could be applied to other state institutions.

Even though the number of counties served by the asylum had been reduced in 1894 to eighteen, the patient population continued to grow and to crowd the institution, and reports of injury to patients by attendants became public. In 1897, an elderly farmer committed to the asylum was injured by an attendant, who was charged with assault. In the incident, the patient's jaw had been broken, his face cut, and his body bruised. The attendant, dismissed from his position, argued that in trying to open the door he had forced it, so the door hit the patient, thus injuring him.[10] Ten years later a young dentist from Parkersburg, West Virginia, staying overnight at the asylum where his father had taken him to spend the night en route to a private sanatorium in Columbus, left with a broken jaw. In 1907, reports of patient injuries and death at the hands of attendants at Athens reached the state's news media.[11] Also that year two patients became pregnant while at the asylum.

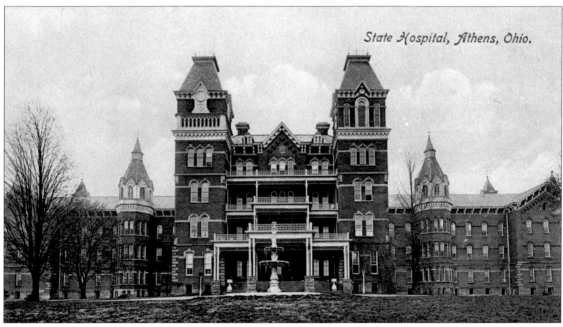

State Hospital, Athens, Ohio.

FIGURE E.1 Postcard showing the front of the building in winter. The photograph was taken after the portico *(center)* was added in 1894. The central administrative section was renamed Lin Hall in 1997; it now houses Ohio University's Kennedy Museum of Art. Renovated patient rooms and wards are now used as studios and gallery space by graduate students in Ohio University's School of Art. *Courtesy of the Mahn Center for Archives and Special Collections, Ohio University Libraries.*

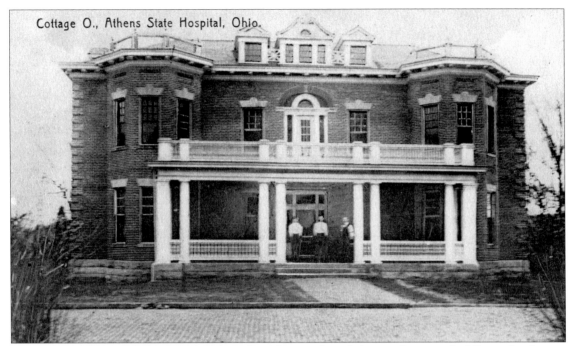

FIGURE E.2 Cottage O, built in 1903 for male patients, reflected the new "cottage plan" form of asylum architecture. The building now houses offices for Ohio University's Voinovich School of Leadership and Public Affairs. *Courtesy of the Mahn Center for Archives and Special Collections, Ohio University Libraries.*

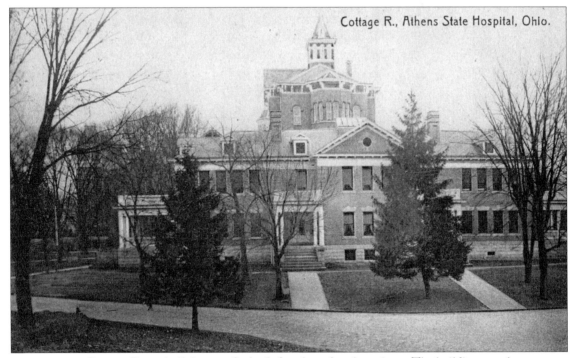

FIGURE E.3 Cottage R was built in 1903 for both female and male patients. The building now houses offices for Ohio University's Voinovich School of Leadership and Public Affairs. *Courtesy of the Mahn Center for Archives and Special Collections, Ohio University Libraries.*

John Wooley, a law student at Ohio State University who was home in Athens for the summer of 1907, obtained work as an attendant at the asylum. Following the death of a patient at the hands of three attendants, Wooley lodged a complaint with the governor about his observation of mistreatment of patients at Athens during the superintendency of Dr. James Hanson. Wrote Mr. Wooley,

> I did not go to the hospital to find out anything, though a cousin of mine is an inmate. I wanted work and went and asked for a place. I was assigned to ward 19, which was considered one of the bad wards. It was in ward 18 that Barnes was killed the other day, and it was in 17 that Cain was killed some years ago. . . . For what were the men beaten? Well, I will give you an instance. There was a patient who was practically an imbecile. When he heard the whistle for meals he knew enough to line up with the others and go to eat, but that was about all. One day, coming back from dinner, he was walking slow. . . . [H]e didn't move fast enough and the attendant kicked him. The kick hurt the attendant's foot and angered him. So he knocked the patient down with a club. . . . [I]t was either fists, clubs or kicks they got: broomsticks, long gas lighters with a ring of rubber on the end, and sticks with . . . cast iron on the sides which were used to clean sink holes. . . . [M]ost of the patients [in 19] were harmless. . . . There was one boy whose head had so many cuts and scars that one could hardly count them. . . . I have seen handles from sweeping brooms broken in several pieces over his head. . . . I saw a man beaten with a club until his body was covered with bruises, stripped of clothes, shut up in the strong room, without supper, to stay all night, with orders to leave him there a week on bread and water (orders from the attendant who beat him). This would have been done, but it was my turn on the ward, and I let him out, under heavy opposition for the other attendant. . . . I saw a perfectly harmless boy, harmless as an infant, knocked from his seat to the floor, kicked by [the] attendant with his heavy shoe many times, stamped in the body, lifted to his seat, grasped by the hair, his head held back with one hand and struck with all force in the face with the other many times. I have seen this same person beaten more than once the same day.[12]

Superintendent Hanson resigned in 1908 after one year of service, and an earlier medical superintendent, Dr. Estell Rorick, returned to hold things together for a year until Ora Otis Fordyce was appointed.

Medical superintendent from 1909 to 1919, Dr. Fordyce led the asylum through several changes. In 1910, Ohio's families were required to pay up to four dollars per week for their relatives' stays in an asylum, a departure from the free care that had previously been provided. A nursing school was established, and in 1911 the asylum graduated its first class of nursing students. In that year also, in an effort to limit political influence over purchasing and jobs in its institutions, the State of Ohio did away with governance by individual boards of trustees. The new system centralized governance in one State Board of Administration, a four-person board of mixed political parties responsible for appointing the heads of all the benevolent and correctional state institutions.

In 1913, the asylum housed on average 1,385 patients on any given day, with a growing number of elderly patients. The wards were crowded with beds closely placed together. Rooms designed for one person housed two or more patients. Wrote Dr. Fordyce, "It is interesting to note that 14% of the admissions [in 1913] were patients suffering from senile psychoses. The growing tendency of sending these old people to our state hospitals partially accounts for the seemingly general increase in insanity. These unfortunate people are suffering from changes incident to old age, are enfeebled and harmless, and most of them should be cared for at home."[13]

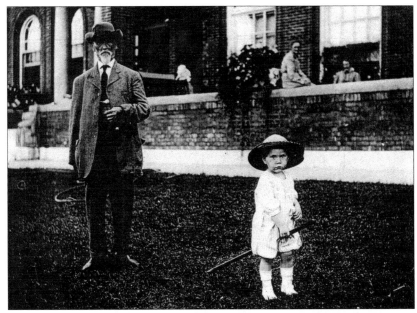

FIGURE E.4 John T. Sprague, son of John Sprague (asylum physician) and Anna Devlyn Sprague, playing on the lawn of the asylum, early twentieth century. *Photograph courtesy of the Athens County Historical Society and Museum Photo Collection.*

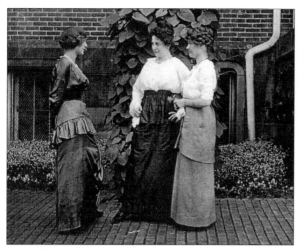

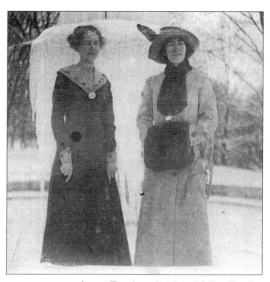

FIGURE E.5 Anna Devlyn *(left)* and May Fordyce *(right)*, wife of Superintendent Fordyce, standing by the frozen fountain in front of the asylum in winter, ca. 1909–19. *Photograph courtesy of the Athens County Historical Society and Museum Photo Collection.*

FIGURE E.6 Asylum nurse Verda Champlin, Mrs. Hughes *(center),* who was the chief nurse, and Mayme Lowell Richardson on the asylum grounds, 1914. *Photograph courtesy of the Athens County Historical Society and Museum Photo Collection.*

FIGURE E.7 Three Athens asylum nurses on asylum grounds, 1911. *Photograph courtesy of the Athens County Historical Society and Museum Photo Collection.*

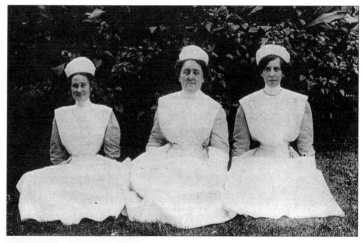

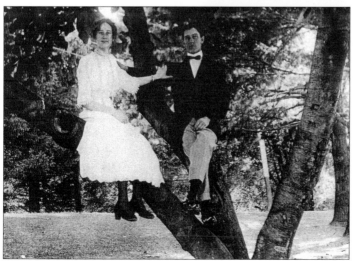

FIGURE E.8 Athens asylum attendants Sadie and Howard Higgins on the asylum grounds, 1913. *Photograph courtesy of the Athens County Historical Society and Museum Photo Collection.*

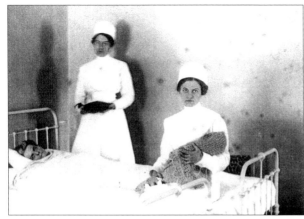

FIGURE E.9 Nurses, patient, and infant at the Athens asylum about 1912. *Photograph courtesy of the Athens County Historical Society and Museum Photo Collection.*

FIGURE E.10 Patients out walking on the Athens asylum grounds, about 1912. *Photograph courtesy of the Athens County Historical Society and Museum Photo Collection.*

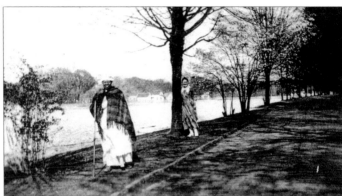

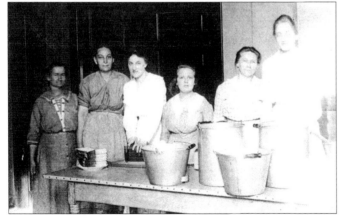

FIGURE E.11 Patients who worked in the asylum kitchen, 1910. *Photograph courtesy of the Athens County Historical Society and Museum Photo Collection.*

FIGURE E.12 Staff and patients who worked in the asylum kitchen, early twentieth century. *Photograph courtesy of the Athens County Historical Society and Museum Photo Collection.*

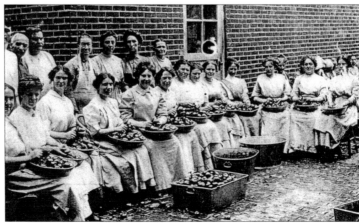

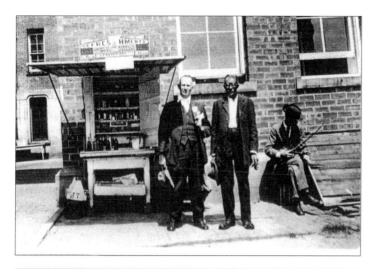

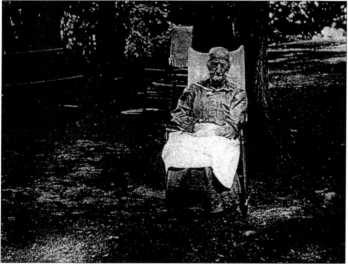

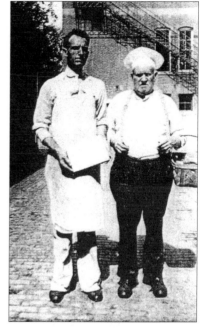

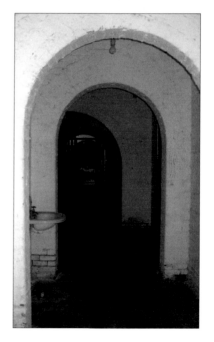

(*from top*) FIGURE E.13 Asylum patients at a refreshment stand to the rear of the asylum, early twentieth century; the patient at right has a violin. *Photograph courtesy of the Athens County Historical Society and Museum Photo Collection.*

FIGURE E.14 Patients who worked as bakers at the asylum, early twentieth century. *Photograph courtesy of the Athens County Historical Society and Museum Photo Collection.*

FIGURE E.15 An elderly patient at the asylum, early twentieth century. *Photograph courtesy of the Athens County Historical Society and Museum Photo Collection.*

FIGURE E.16 Unrenovated section of basement. *Photograph courtesy of Doug McCabe.*

At asylums across the United States, patient populations grew far beyond the several hundred recommended by moral treatment psychiatry, some to extremes. Milledgeville asylum in Georgia in the early twentieth century, for example, had grown to hold more than ten thousand patients.[14]

Treatment in the first quarter of the twentieth century consisted mainly of employment (giving patients work to do), amusement, and hydrotherapy. As early as 1800, physicians in Europe had applied newly developed technologies of the Industrial Revolution to psychiatric treatments involving water. At that time, asylum doctors used bizarre water treatments such as jets of cold water to the head, hidden trapdoors through which patients would plunge for a "bath of surprise," and coffins with holes drilled in them into which patients were put and held underwater—the shock of near-drowning was thought to have a curative effect.[15] By the early twentieth century, hydrotherapy in America's asylums had evolved into widely used and somewhat more sedate treatments used to calm patient behaviors. Treatments included fomentations (hot and cold compresses applied alternately) and Scotch douches (alternating warm and cold needle showers). Patients receiving wet sheet packs were wrapped for several hours in sheets that had been soaked in cold water and wrung out. Salt glows were salt and oil scrubs. Athens superintendent Dr. Fordyce wrote in 1913, "I regard hydrotherapy of great importance in treating the insane. Its use has allowed us to practically eliminate hypnotics and mechanical restraints. Patients are more quiet and better contented. It gives relief to many painful mental states, quiets the noisy, avoids complications, retards dementia and I verily believe increases the percentage of recoveries."[16] At Athens in 1914, 6,413 hydrotherapy treatments were administered to 246 women; 8,041 treatments were administered to 165 men (see table E. 1). Hydrotherapy remained a treatment staple well into midcentury, with nearly 5,000 wet sheet packs and 2,156 continuous baths administered in 1953.

Beyond hydrotherapy, asylum physicians continued to rely on amusements and useful occupation to keep patients' minds and bodies busy. Wrote Dr. Fordyce,

> Occupation is now recognized as one of the princip[a]l methods of treating the insane. I observe that when patients are wholesomely employed, several hours daily, there is but little, if any, mental deterioration. It is the patients who sit idly on the wards that dement. . . . Systematic occupation

TABLE E.1
Hydrotherapy treatments in 1914
(combined total of 14,454)

Treatment	Number of treatments administered	
	Men	Women
Continuous baths	1,173	547
Electric cabinet	438	97
Fomentations	101	15
Needle sprays	26	2,069
Salt glows	1,888	1,972
Sprays and Scotch douches	3,957	1,129
Wet sheet packs	458	584
Total number of treatments	8,041	6,413
Number of patients treated	165	246

Source: Thirty-Ninth Report of the Athens State Hospital for the Year Ending November 15, 1914 to the Ohio Board of Administration (Athens, 1914).

will train the hand and enliven the brain to act in harmony, and by this gentle stimulation, aid in restoring mental equilibrium. I am a great believer in the therapeutic potency of occupation, and it is the policy of the hospital to have something for every able-bodied patient to do.[17]

Toward this end, the asylum at Athens through the 1930s offered handwork such as the making of baskets, rugs, and paper flowers; dances for patients with music by the asylum's own eight-piece orchestra; a Victrola; and holiday celebrations. Superintendent Fordyce described the systematic occupation:

[P]atients are employed in a well lighted, attractive room from 8 to 11 A.M., and from 1 to 4 P.M., every week day except Saturday afternoon. Special inducements are offered in the way of refreshments, music, etc., in order to make the work as inviting and interesting as possible. The work and personal influence of the teacher, supported by the interest and enthusiasm on the part of the more active patients . . . becomes contagious . . . to the disinclined patients. Many of them will become interested in something they see others doing, and with careful training and patience, may be taught to become useful, and thereby arrest the progress of mental decay.[18]

Patients worked in the asylum's sewing room, kitchens, dairy and livestock operations, and gardens. If patients could not provide useful work in their homes and communities and contribute to the prosperity of their families, some patients found their work in the asylum meaningful and fulfilling. Certainly their work contributed to the operation of the asylum. The economy of the institution at Athens and at state asylums nationwide in the first half of the twentieth century became dependent on the labor of their patients, supporting a system in which physicians and their families (who lived on-site) enjoyed privilege in exchange for overseeing care of the patients, many of whom farmed and performed other essential services. Male patients worked on the asylum farms, which produced abundant harvests of fruits and vegetables as well as dairy products and meats. Superintendent John Berry wrote a history of the asylum in 1926 for the Ohio Department of Public Welfare, providing a sketch of its landscape and farming operations.

> [It is] not an "Asylum" but a modern, up-to-date State Hospital for the care and treatment of the insane. It is a little city in itself, being located in the midst of a beautiful park of more than 60 acres. The charm of which is due to the artist who planned it many years ago and to those who cared for and improved it in years gone by. The Institution now has a farm of over one thousand acres. Eighty acres in garden, acres of well kept, thrifty orchards and vineyards. It has one of the finest Holstein dairy herds in the State. Instead of purchasing milk and butter, as was the practice in the early days, this dairy produced last year sufficient milk and butter for the needs of the Institution to the value of $32,192.88. The Institution has a population of 1500—175 of whom are employees. The farm, dairy, garden, orchard and other activities not only are utilized to make the Institution more nearly self-supporting but to provide healthful occupation for the patients coming to it for treatment.[19]

Dr. Berry continued his history with a description of the asylum's medical treatment facilities. "The Institution is now equipped with an X-Ray outfit, hydrotherapy, modern dental office, laboratory and operating room. This equipment together with the modern day knowledge of mental and nervous disease enables the Institution to cure a greater percentage of patients than was possible years ago." In 1924, Cottage B was built to house up to

150 patients with tuberculosis. Constructed of brick and concrete and located above the fog line, it featured sleeping porches for sun treatments and large windows for sunlight and airflow.

In the 1950s, some asylum superintendents and physicians felt they were impeded in their efforts to provide up-to-date therapy because of institutional structures and traditions that had been in place for decades.[20] A critique of asylum culture presented at the annual meeting of the American Psychiatric Association in 1948 by Columbus (Ohio) State Hospital superintendent J. Fremont Bateman suggested that a dual cultural system existed in state mental hospitals. Bateman believed that the therapeutic goals of physicians were at odds with the structures, power, roles, and status of hospital staff. Most superintendents, he noted, were unwilling at that time to take the risks required to make systemic changes. At that time, asylum staff governed the daily routines, rewards, assignments, and freedom of patients; patients in turn discussed among themselves and competed for certain things, chief among which was going home, with others being assignment to a certain ward or a certain job, the attentions of physicians, and the good-will of attendants.

At Athens in the mid-twentieth century, 413 employees, about half of whom were attendants, were on the payroll. Four physicians, a psychologist, a psychology assistant, a psychiatric social worker, and a recreational therapist directed patient treatment. The pharmacy, known as the Drug Room, was staffed by an attendant. The last of the major architectural additions to the asylum complex had been completed. In 1950, a 45,000-square-foot general hospital was constructed; the following year, two brick buildings were completed for physicians' living quarters, followed by a new laundry and an 8,000-square-foot power plant. The old greenhouse was razed in 1953.

Desperate to relieve and control the symptoms of their patients, by the late 1940s American asylum physicians were employing new treatments: ECT (electroconvulsive therapy or electric shock therapy, as it was called then) and, for a short time, psychosurgery (lobotomies), both of which were performed at Athens in its new hospital. Dr. Walter Freeman, who traveled the nation giving the transorbital "ice-pick" variety of lobotomy at state asylums, visited the asylum at Athens twice a year for several years.[21] His last visit was on May 7, 1956, on which day he performed twenty-nine lobotomies. The transorbital lobotomy was performed under ECT anesthesia. That is, a patient was administered ECT and during the short period of unconsciousness following received the lobotomy. In 1953, staff at Athens performed thirty-nine lobotomies and administered electric shock therapy to 195 patients for a total of 2,914 treatments. The asylum's lobotomy experience was summarized by Hubert Haymond Fockler (superintendent, 1955–62).[22]

> We have been doing lobotomies here at Athens for several
> years and several hundreds of them have been done. The
> transorbital, pre-frontal and for the past four years the
> Dr. Walter Freeman type of transorbital lobotomy. Dr.
> Freeman introduced lobotomy into America following the
> original work of E. Moniz in Portugal. The earlier type
> of lobotomy was not so effective. The more recent type is
> more curative in our experience.
>
> The attempt in psychosurgery of all types is to sever
> fibers connecting the thalamus (emotions, feelings) with
> the cortex (acting, responses). The operation is not without
> some risk, therefore, it is not resorted to until other
> methods of treatment such as ECT, tranquilizing drugs
> or routine therapy [have] failed to bring about a cure. Our
> results from this procedure have been quite encouraging
> considering the type and number of patients that have
> been able to remain out of the Hospital.
>
> Dr. Freeman comes twice a year for a series of
> operations. He did not come this fall due to making a trip
> to England to address the Royal society on twenty years of
> Leucotomy [another name for the lobotomy].
>
> We have done to date 208 transorbital lobotomies on
> 192 patients. A few patients had the second operation.
>
> The mortality rate from this operation has been given
> as from two to five per cent. In the last 55 operations
> we have had one death due to fatal hemorrhage. The
> technique is rather simple. The operation is done under
> ECT anaesthesia. Of 208 operations performed on 192
> patients, 116 patients are still out of the Hospital.
>
> Before the operation is done Dr. Freeman usually talks
> to the families of the patients, in a group, explaining the
> operation and the after management of the patient. He
> examines each patient and makes a summary, indicating the
> reasons for lobotomy and giving a pre-operative prognosis.

> As stated we have not done any operations since last May 7th. On that date 29 cases were operated with no deaths. [They were] unfavorable cases who had had other methods of treatment without response. 18 of these 29 are at home today; that is about 60%, and 60% is about the rate of remissions over the four years that we have been doing this type of operations.[23]

In 1953, into the midst of lobotomies, electroconvulsive therapy, hydrotherapy, and employment on the farms and in the sewing rooms, was introduced a program of birthday parties for patients.

> For many years it was the dream of Mrs. Creed, our Superintendent's wife, that each patient should have a Birthday party. In January of this year we started having parties on the third and fourth Thursdays of each month, a party for each patient having a birthday in that particular month. This is a Gray Lady [Red Cross volunteer] assignment and we always have several Gray ladies to help with the entertainment. We try to have a variety of games so that all can participate. Also group singing and story telling by the patients themselves are very popular. We have ice cream and cake with each patient receiving a piece of cake with a candle. Those who are bed patients or are unable to attend are sent refreshments on the ward.[24]

American asylums reached their peak populations in the 1950s. At Athens, the average daily population in 1953 was 1,747. Wrote Superintendent Creed that year, "[W]e were so over crowded, especially with old folks, that we had no place to transfer [newly admitted patients] from the Receiving Building, so that it was necessary to suspend accepting voluntary admission."[25] Dr. Creed hired staff that year to expand the range of services. A recreational therapist began a music therapy program staffed by faculty and students from Ohio University. Among other projects, the music therapists played recorded music for patients waiting for electric shock treatments to ease their fear and anxiety about the procedure. After some experimentation, the right kind of music was found. Charlotte Cox, recreational therapist, reported on the results of that project: "At first light classical selections were played. When the record selection was changed, the lighter movements of symphonies were tried. Symphonic music was totally unfamiliar to the patients and they complained that this type [of] music was depressing to them. They requested Hillbilly and popular music. At present Bing Crosby records are being played and there have not been any complaints thus far."[26] Dr. Creed also hired a psychiatric social service supervisor to supervise the care of patients on trial home visits and to coordinate care with families as well as psychologists to assess patients upon arrival and administer a wide variety of psychological tests.[27]

Meanwhile the asylum's farming operations, worked by employees and patients, boomed. The agricultural program was important enough to be listed in the 1953 annual report as one of the three principal functions of the asylum, in addition to the treatment and care of patients with mental disorders and the giving of psychiatric advice to patients not admitted to the hospital. Nearly 17,000 gallons of vegetables and fruits were canned that year by the kitchen staff with the help of patients. Their work included the canning of green beans, beets, pumpkin, various kinds of relish, rhubarb, tomatoes, peas, and pickles. The asylum's hens laid 26,227 dozen eggs, its dairying operation yielded over a million gallons of milk and nearly 17,000 pounds of butter; 118,124 pounds of pork were produced; and tons of silage, fodder, and hay were grown. Fresh fruits and vegetables from the farm abounded: in 1953, the kitchens prepared and served 103,000 pounds of cabbage, 17,888 pounds of lima beans, 12,000 pounds of onions, 111,825 pounds of sweet corn in the husk, and a quarter of a million pounds of apples from the farm. The bounty of the farming operation was varied: broccoli, beets, Brussels sprouts, cauliflower, cabbage, eggplant, horseradish, kale, lettuces, okra, parsley, parsnips, popcorn, sweet potatoes, radishes, rhubarb, sage, squash, Swiss chard, turnips, watermelon, peanuts, strawberries, peaches, and grapes. Honey was also collected. The garden production lasted another fifteen years before it began to decline.

Deinstitutionalization

By 1968 with the national deinstitutionalization movement well under way, the asylum at Athens had begun to reduce its number of patients. Deinstitutionalization, the relocating of asylum patients to their communities, was a result of several factors, including the rise of new models of care from treatment lessons learned in World War II; the 1963 Community Mental Health Act; the availability of a new, wide range of medications; the influence of the antipsychiatry/asylum reform movement; and the 1973 patient labor court decision, which essentially eliminated patient work programs at most state hospitals. In the European theater in World War II, American physicians learned that their patients recovered more quickly when they were treated at field hospitals near their units rather than in distant hospitals. This learning informed the work of the Joint Commission on Mental Illness and Mental Health established by Congress in 1955. The commission recommended a new system of community-based mental health care, which in turn resulted in the 1963 Community Mental Health Act. Biological psychiatry—medications—radically changed the landscape of patient treatment in the 1960s. Antipsychotic medications such as Thorazine (which reduced the symptoms of psychoses and schizophrenia) along with mood stabilizers (which alleviated the symptoms of bipolar disorder) rendered traditional asylum-based methods of care—hydrotherapy, lobotomies, and physical restraint—obsolete. Chlorpromazine, marketed as Thorazine by Smith-Kline and French, was approved by the U.S. Food and Drug Administration for psychiatric treatment in 1954.[28] At the same time, various components of a powerful antipsychiatry movement had combined to form a critique of asylums. Psychiatrist Thomas Szasz, in his book *The Myth of Mental Illness* (1960), criticized the scientific basis of psychiatry and rejected the existence of mental illness. Sociologist Erving Goffman, in his 1961 book *Asylums: Essays on the Condition of the Social Situation of Mental Patients and Other Inmates,* portrayed mental hospitals as humiliating institutions designed to eradicate the identity of the individual.[29] The film *The Snake Pit* (1948) and Ken Kesey's novel *One Flew Over the Cuckoo's Nest* (1962) contributed to public and political outrage about the state of America's asylums.

Accounts of employees at state asylums in the 1960s portray a sometimes shocking lack of resources and order. Angelina Szot's account of her work as a nurse at Danvers State Hospital in Massachusetts described the lack of clothing and sometimes naked condition of patients.[30] Athens also had problems with laundry and clothing in the 1960s. Harry Chovnick described the laundry situation he encountered when he became superintendent in 1967, with 1,250 patients being cared for by 600 employees:

> In those days clothing was pulled from a pile. The
> laundries were monstrously inefficient in the systems about

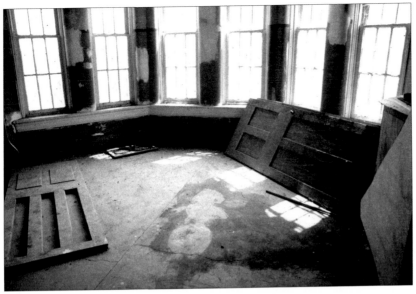

FIGURE E.17 A stain on the floor of one of the patient wings thought to be the form of a female patient found deceased in an abandoned part of the asylum on January 11, 1979; the patient had been missing since December 1, 1978. Analysis of the stain in 2008 by Ohio University researchers suggests that the stain was formed by fatty acids produced by the decomposing body combined with a phosphoric acid-based cleaning fluid. *Photograph courtesy of George Eberts. Originally published in Zimmerman, Laskay, and Jackson, "Analysis of Suspected Trace Human Remains."*

the country. . . . [T]o keep track of clothing was irritating work. Two or three times a week, clothing changes became necessary. . . . [T]he staff and the patients would go through the pile of stuff in the middle of the ward and try to pick out a pair of socks that fit them—not necessarily the same color. Many of them walked around with pants up to mid-shins. They looked like freaks. And others wore pants so long that they dragged.[31]

Finally, the 1973 court decision in *Souder v. Brennan* found that minimum wage and overtime pay applied to patient workers at nonfederal hospitals and institutions for persons with mental illness. State governments across the country were either unwilling or unable to compensate patients for their work in their state mental hospitals, which effectively eliminated patient work programs. For some patients, the loss of the opportunity to work was difficult, even resulting sometimes in suicide attempts. For these patients, their commitment to a personal work ethic made their asylum jobs a point of honor; others found the routine physical activity soothing.[32] In any case, with the economy of state mental hospitals across the nation dependent on the labor of their patients to run the farms, kitchens, laundries, and workshops, the hospitals could no longer make financial ends meet.

During the 1970s and 1980s, the asylum at Athens reduced its patient population from approximately 1,800 patients in 1966 to 200 in 1985. Athens began deinstitutionalization earlier than most

FIGURE E.18 (*right*) Fountain in storage behind the asylum. *Photograph courtesy of Matthew Ziff.*

FIGURE E.19 (*below*) Children's Garden at the Ohio University Child Development Center. The center is located in the newly renovated asylum stables. *Photograph courtesy of Matthew Ziff.*

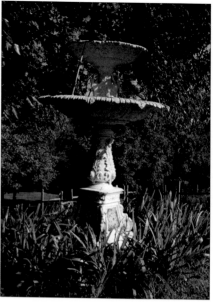

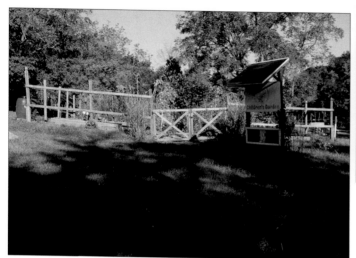

FIGURE E.20 Community recreation golf facility on the asylum grounds. *Photograph courtesy of Matthew Ziff.*

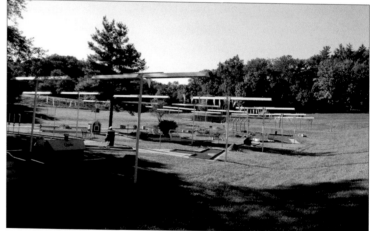

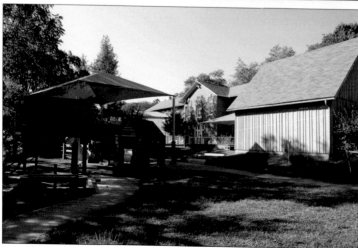

FIGURE E.21 Ohio University Child Development Center, formerly the asylum stables. *Photograph courtesy of Matthew Ziff.*

state hospitals, with the quiet work of Superintendent Gordon Ogram (1964–67).[33] Dr. Sue Foster, who became superintendent at Athens in 1977, continued this work under the direction of the Ohio Department of Mental Health. Staff worked to find suitable places for patients in the community: nursing homes, group homes, subsidized housing, intensive case management, and families. The hospital's social workers identified or created community options for patients and their families. Meanwhile, the asylum continued to provide care for new admissions in its acute and intensive care unit, staffed by a treatment team of psychologists, social workers, a psychiatrist, a psychiatric nurse, ward staff, and trainees.[34] Because of its proximity to Ohio University, the asylum, which had been renamed the Athens Mental Health Center, had become a training institution. Students in the departments of psychology, social work, art therapy, and music therapy as well as the medical school trained at the center, giving the center an energy and leading edge that made it different from some other state hospitals.[35]

For twenty years, Athens asylum superintendents beginning with Dr. David Caul in 1973 had asked for a new, modern hospital. In 1993 their vision was accomplished: the last few patients "came down from the hill" to a new and much smaller state mental hospital just across the Hocking River, leaving the old asylum empty. The new hospital, now known as Appalachian Behavioral Healthcare, is built of brick and features the design of the iron window grilles of the old asylum.

Sixteen years earlier, asylum furnishings dating from the nineteenth century had been dispersed throughout the community through a public auction.[36] Items no longer being used, such as the asylum's original telephone switchboard, rolltop desks, glassware from the officers' dining room, and masses of furniture, were sold at auction in 1977. Through an act of the state legislature, reminiscent of the legislative act transferring the Coates farm to the State of Ohio for the new asylum more than a century previous, the asylum buildings and seven hundred acres were conveyed to Ohio University. The transaction began in 1985 and was completed in 1988. In a community contest sponsored by the university, the complex was renamed The Ridges to reflect the topography of the line of steep hills on which the complex sits. The move left Ohio University with a vast complex of historically and architecturally significant empty buildings and an extensive and varied landscape.

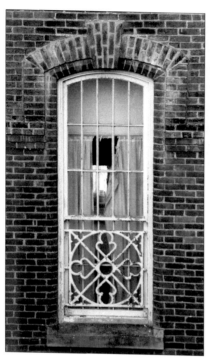

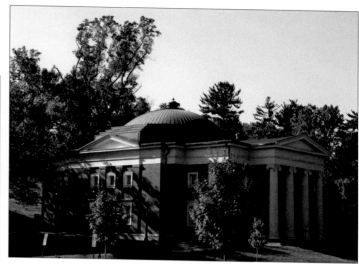

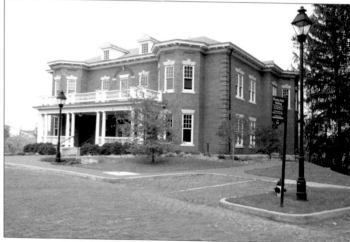

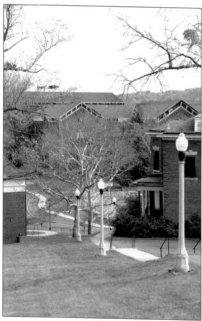

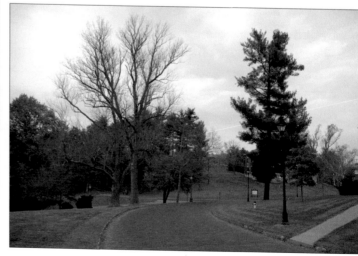

As the immense Victorian buildings of America's state asylums emptied, most were left abandoned. Over three dozen have been demolished, with the pace of demolition quickening in the twenty-first century. Others are untended and have deteriorated beyond reuse. Some—including St. Elizabeths in Washington, Fergus Falls in Minnesota, Taunton State Hospital in Massachusetts, and the Hudson River State Hospital in New York—have suffered fires and are either empty or demolished. The remaining Kirkbride asylum buildings are substantial architectural records of the 150-year story of the history of American asylumdom; first the original Kirkbride central buildings, then the introduction of residential cottages at the turn of the century, and finally in the 1950s the additions of a geriatric clinic, the general hospital, and other clinics to serve the needs of patients. These remaining asylums are also a record of the vernacular architecture, materials, and construction of their communities and regions.[37] Some continue to operate as mental health centers or prisons. A few, such as Traverse City State Hospital in Michigan and Greystone Park in New Jersey, are supported by private, community, or state government groups that have begun work to preserve their historical buildings and landscapes.[38]

The Athens asylum on The Ridges is one of a small handful of American Kirkbride asylum buildings that have been successfully repurposed—one might argue that it is the most advanced example. The preservation of the complex at Athens has evolved over several decades "through the efforts of planners, architects, landscape architects and administrators who preserved the old,

(*opposite, from top*) FIGURE E.22 Amusement hall, built in 1900. Today it is used for university and community events and classes. *Photograph courtesy of Matthew Ziff.*

FIGURE E.23 Window in unrenovated portion of the original building. *Photograph courtesy of Matthew Ziff.*

FIGURE E.24 Cottage R, built in 1903 as living quarters for male and females, as it appears in 2011, renovated to house university offices. *Photograph courtesy of Matthew Ziff.*

FIGURE E.25 View of Cottage M, built in 1903 (*right foreground*), and original Kirkbride buildings (*background*). *Photograph courtesy of Matthew Ziff.*

FIGURE E.26 Brick drive and landscape encircling the main asylum complex. *Photograph courtesy of Matthew Ziff.*

created the new, and in the process became guardians and curators of the distinct character of the site."[39]

Even while the asylum at Athens continued to serve patients, it was evolving into a new existence. Its repurposing has featured planning, consideration of an array of uses, many community discussions, public tours, political deals, money, and the university architects, planners, and project managers who have been stewards of the buildings and their landscape of open space. The first significant renovation project was undertaken by the Athens community in 1977 when the asylum's dairy complex was scheduled to be demolished. One of the barns was saved by the work of a citizens' task force headed by artist Harriet Anderson and her husband, Ora. With nine days to spare, the task force and the Hocking Valley Arts Council succeeded in petitioning the governor to preserve the barn, now known as The Dairy Barn Arts Center, a nonprofit organization.[40] By 1981, the Athens community had geared up to discuss renovation and reuse of the enormous complex on the hill. A volunteer nonprofit organization, the Athens County Urban Redevelopment Corporation, hoped to sublease the property to private developers for a research park, a retirement center, a conference center, a golf course, or other uses. None came to pass—to the especial disappointment of Athens residents working toward a retirement center renovation. Shortly thereafter, Ohio University began to study possibilities for a research park on the site and then commissioned a comprehensive land-use study published in 1989.

The complex is vast, containing 707,437 gross square feet, with 225,813 net square feet of space now renovated or retrofitted and assigned to forty-five specific university uses. They include a child development center in the newly renovated horse barn; the auditorium built in 1901, which has been renovated and is used for university and community events and classes; geology and geography research; and the Ohio University Press. The Kennedy Museum of Art, with its galleries and studio space, occupies the central Kirkbride administrative section of the complex; its plaster and tile interiors gleam with the patina of history and fresh paint. The old kitchens and bake shop are now used for university service functions such as mail and surplus property. Graduate art students use as studio and exhibition space the renovated third floor of the original wing for male patients. Cottage

R, built for male and female patients in 1903, has been renovated and houses the Voinovich School of Leadership and Public Affairs. Cottage L, built in 1909, houses the Edison Biotechnology Institute.

The location of the biotechnology institute was the subject of controversy in the early 1990s. The university originally proposed a new building on the top of the high ground in the midst of the seven hundred acres of open space known as Radar Hill. In the 1960s and 1970s, that site featured a laboratory run by the Department of Electrical Engineering's Avionics program, which included several radar dishes, antennae, and transmitters located there by arrangement with the asylum. Computer work was done on the main campus, and the results were hand-carried up to the laboratory.[41] At the request of faculty and chairs of departments including botany and zoology, the Radar Hill site remained open space for land lab research and teaching, and the biotechnology center location was moved to Cottage L. Ohio University botany (now environmental and plant biology) professor Phillip D. Cantino noted at the time, in reference to the open space, "Very few [universities] have a jewel like this on their doorstep."[42]

Renovating and repurposing the buildings have been accomplished with the factors of money, timing, and building function coming together at the right time, as Ohio University emerged as the only entity in rural southeastern Ohio able to fully assume responsibility for the development of the seven hundred acres of open space plus thirty acres of buildings. Many developers with plans for retirement housing and other commercial and residential uses have made preliminary investigations for adaptive reuse, but none have been realized.

The principal challenge to repurposing has been cost, including the potential assumption by the university of debt service on behalf of private developers. The buildings' massive and sturdy load-bearing masonry construction does not lend itself to inexpensive renovation. In contrast to modern buildings held up with structures of steel beams and columns filled in with wall and mechanical systems that can be relatively easily moved, the asylum's spaces are less flexible. The building is supported by stone and brick walls two and three feet thick at the building's base. The interior walls of the hallways and patient rooms are also thick, heavy brick load-bearing structures. The floor joists, made of heavy timber of relatively short length, perhaps ten to twenty feet long, require frequent load-bearing masonry walls. These walls must be painstakingly removed with jackhammers and picks while the structure is carefully supported and reinforced as modern mechanical systems are added. As with most old buildings, lead paint and asbestos cleanup is a consideration. Another challenge has been the perception of separation of the asylum complex from the main Ohio University campus by the Hocking River and by topography—the steep ridge on which the buildings sit.[43]

Despite the challenges, the successes are many. With privately developed student housing extending behind the asylum complex, The Ridges is no longer at the edge of the developed part of town and campus. A new road system with a pedestrian tunnel and an improved bridge has created ease of access. Also, buildings on asylum land transferred to local government agencies as part of the conveyance of the property to the university have been renovated and are thriving as the Dairy Barn Regional Art Center, the university's Eco House, the local mental health board, and a municipal recreation complex with a baseball field, miniature golf facility, and picnic shelter.

Ohio University now owns of one of the best-preserved Kirkbride asylums in America. The 2001 Architectural Master Plan evaluated all the buildings of the former asylum campus for the historical significance of their exterior architecture and determined whether each was of primary, secondary, or tertiary significance; this document provides preservation guidelines based on the exterior architectural significance of the buildings. Of primary significance are the original Kirkbride building and the cottages structures added in the early 1900s. Although the latest campus master plan (2006) gives permission to demolish the outer wings of the original building should a better use be found, the plan recommends in any case preserving the original "thunderbird" shape with its central administrative area and the first wing on each side, as well as the existing cottage plan buildings already renovated.[44] The Kennedy Museum, with its two floors of renovated gallery and studio space, firmly anchors this original building. The challenge to further renovation and reuse is, of course, finding funds to do the work. The asylum is a hardy, robust building by nature of its masonry construction, and with some help in protecting the roof and window openings to keep water out and the masonry and building structurally sound, it could last another 150 years. The university has demonstrated a commitment to this end, with a program of replacing in 2009 half of the roof of the original building. With its commitment to renovation and repurposing, the university has preserved a remarkable set of buildings with local as well as national architectural, cultural, and historical significance.

In addition to the buildings of the old asylum, Ohio University is steward to seven hundred acres of open space. The comprehensive land use study of The Ridges published in 1989 (which inventoried and assessed the entire site as well as the buildings) sought comments and advice from the Athens community. The Ridges Advisory Committee member Ora Anderson described the state of the land in 1988:

> As far as the land is concerned, some of the most
> beautiful land that we've got left in the [Athens] area
> is located up there and it is of all kinds: heavily wooded
> areas that are old woods, small planted woodlands
> that goes back to about 1930, open fields, pasture lands
> and meadow lands, the old orchard which is now a
> brushland, it's got everything up there that you can
> think of that any out doors people might like. And so
> that too is going to require . . . an approach . . . that is
> gradual rather than sudden. . . . [W]e can use physical
> judgments in some instances to decide the future of
> some land but we have to determine others on the
> basis of ecological values, educational values, as well as
> economic values."[45]

Anderson's comments echo those of Dr. Richard Gundry in his 1872 report to the asylum's board of trustees.

In the fall of 2000, the oldest of the three patient cemeteries at the asylum at Athens was featured on a national television program about the world's scariest places. Appalled at the stigma such exposure brought to mental illness, people from the local Alcohol, Drug Addiction, and Mental Health Services Board, the Ohio Department of Mental Health, the National Alliance for Mental Illness, Ohio University, The Gathering Place, the Civilian Conservation Corps, and others mobilized to form the Ridges Cemeteries

Committee to clean up and restore the cemeteries. Today the cemeteries and their landscape are restored and connected by a nature walk featuring regenerated forests and ecodiversity.[46] The seven hundred acres of open space also feature a challenge course used by university classes and community organizations, ROTC practice areas, nature trails, and many acres used for land lab research and teaching.

The asylum exists vividly today in the community memories of family and friends who were employees or patients or relatives of the same. Many persons in the Athens community hold memories and convictions about the asylum and the land. Some still remember the alligator that lived in the fountain in front of the asylum in the summer months, the bequest of an employee who brought back a baby alligator from a trip to Florida. Former employees recall the camaraderie of apple picking, quiet winter nights working on the wards overlooking newly fallen snow, and picnic dinners. Athenians remember sledding on the hillsides and ice skating on the old lakes. Families of patients recall days of loss and confusion mixed with hope as they sought help for their children or parents. A legacy of stigma still clings, taking form in persistent undocumented tales. University students speculate about ghosts of former patients haunting the spaces, their imaginations inspired by the immense building with its towers and stairs. The interior spaces, especially the unrenovated floors of the original Kirkbride building and cottages, remain layered with nearly a century and a half of memories. They are tempered, though, by the hope and care suggested by sunlight that streams through the tall iron-grilled windows and illuminates the spaces.

Ohio University's work at renovating and repurposing the massive brick buildings to accommodate a range of activities hints at the asylum's beginning as a site for humane, moral treatment of mental illness that drew upon nature, the arts, families, politics, and community for healing its patients. Today the Kirkbride building and the Colonial Revival–style cottages and their grounds host university-based operations for child care, environmental studies, medical research, art education, and publishing. The architectural centerpiece, the Kirkbride High Victorian Italianate central administrative core, now houses an art museum. Vestiges of the original landscape remain—a stone wall here, an old apple tree there, a once-grand fountain now preserved in storage. The grounds today are devoted to nature trails, a land lab, forests, creeks, and fields and are the delight of hikers and Sunday afternoon strollers in all seasons and weather. With its apple trees, blackberry hedges, plum thickets, forests, meadows, spring wildflowers, milkweed, sycamore trees, hawks, wild turkeys, bluebirds, deer, and monarch butterflies, The Ridges is a modern-day asylum, or sanctuary, for restoration of tranquility and health.

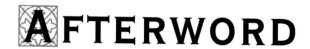

AFTERWORD

to the 150th Anniversary Edition

The epilogue of *Asylum on the Hill* describes many of challenges and successes that have emerged in the adaptive reuse of this property following its transfer to Ohio University. One aspect that remains the same, though, is the strong sense of connection that many members of the community feel with this distinctive place, with its striking architecture and engaging landscape adjacent to and increasingly entwined with the city of Athens. However, portions of the buildings have stood unoccupied for more than three decades, and although a variety of uses have been suggested for the land, the future of what we now call The Ridges has lingered on as a question.

A new piece of this story emerged with the completion in 2016 of The Ridges Framework Plan, developed by the university in close partnership with members of the community. Several previous studies had evaluated the potential for adaptive reuse of the buildings and outdoor space, in some cases with a specific outcome in mind. The Framework Plan began with a broad examination of the suitability and compatibility of the buildings and land for a diverse range of outcomes. The analysis is distinctive in pointing to a mix of sustainable uses, evoking the linkage of the built and natural environments that supported the original mission of the asylum. The result of this process is a flexible scheme that confirms the integrity and adaptability of the buildings for a wide range of purposes; acknowledges a hierarchy of value for the buildings that informs priorities for preservation; and envisions multiple potential uses for the land, with much of it to remain in a natural state.

The Framework Plan acknowledges the compelling role of architecture and landscape in defining a unique sense of place and a connection to history at The Ridges. Any visitor gazing at the imposing Victorian structure and its adjacent cemeteries and woods invariably asks, *What is this place and why is it here?* The Ridges provides a unique asset for learning about the history of public engagement with mental illness in America, encapsulating in built form and tranquil landscapes the philosophy of moral treatment and its successors. The facility also embodies the optimism of the nineteenth century in establishing institutions, including asylums and universities, to benefit society.

The conversation involved in creating the Framework Plan and follow-on developments has brought renewed interest in the asylum. The collaborative approach to planning and the resulting buy-in from interested parties has helped motivate new investments from the university to benefit both campus and community. Stabilization work has been completed to prevent water intrusion in the buildings, and eroded stonework has been rebuilt on the asylum portico and elsewhere. The grounds host a new astronomical observatory, and an expansion of the Kennedy Museum has begun. Coincident with the sesquicentennial of the asylum's founding, Ohio University is moving forward with a major renovation that will lead to adaptive reuse of half of the original Kirkbride wings for office space. These activities will complement the academic endeavors already ongoing elsewhere at The Ridges.

These developments since the original publication of *Asylum on the Hill* can be seen as a heightened affirmation of Ohio University's embrace of this facility and of the value of distinctive places to advance the public good. The Ridges' adaptive reuse brings new life and vitality to these spaces and the community, while respecting the historic legacy of patients and caregivers engaged in moral treatment.

Shawna Bolin and Joseph C. Shields
Ohio University
April 2018

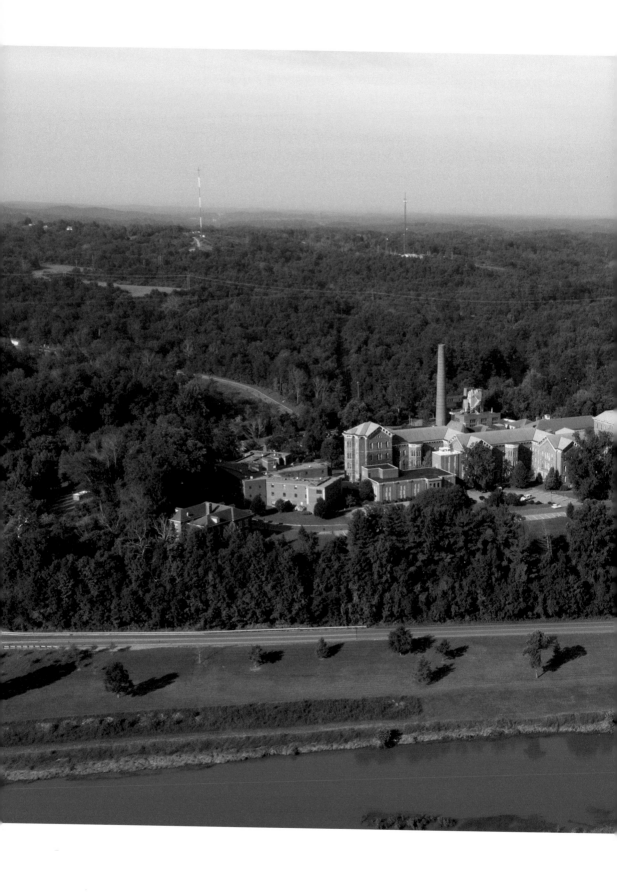

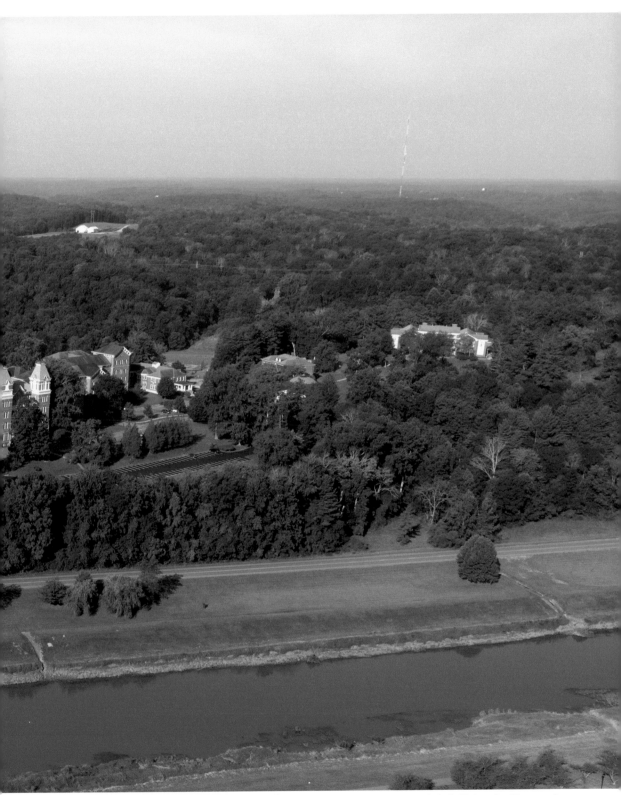

Aerial photograph of The Ridges, summer of 2017. *Photograph by Ben Siegel, © Ohio University Photography*

NOTES

Preface

1. The mounds may also have served as a means of communication among these Late Woodland period tribes. See Eliot Abrams and AnnCorinne Freter's edited volume *The Emergence of the Moundbuilders: The Archaeology of Tribal Societies in Southeastern Ohio* (Athens: Ohio University Press, 2005) for a modern interpretation of the indigenous societies of the Ohio Valley.

2. See Andrew Scull, "Psychiatry and Social Control in the Nineteenth and Twentieth Centuries," *History of Psychiatry* 2 (1991): 149–69, in which Scull states, "My own view is that both these perspectives are too crude and one-sided. In its origins, at least, nineteenth-century lunacy reform was Janus-faced; simultaneously embodying (at least at the outset) 'a humanitarian concern for the protection, against visible abuses, of people who were coming to be seen as curable sufferers whose condition was not their fault'; while (to some degree unwittingly) fostering a concealed yet ever more systematic regulation of lunatics' lives . . . only over time were these tensions (repression vs. rehabilitation) systematically resolved in favour of an oppressive system of moral management, enforced conformity, and disciplined subordination" (153–54).

3. For a detailed discussion of a taxonomy of therapeutic places, see Fiona Smyth, "Medical Geography: Therapeutic Places, Spaces and Networks," *Progress in Human Geography* 29 (2005): 488–95. For photographs and descriptions of American Kirkbride hospitals and their landscapes, see www.kirkbridebuildings.com.

4. Witold Rybczynski, *A Clearing in the Distance: Frederick Law Olmsted and America in the Nineteenth Century* (New York: Scribner, 1999).

5. Esther M. Sternberg, *Healing Spaces: The Science of Place and Well-Being* (Cambridge, MA: Belknap Press, 2009). Sternberg describes a period when Jonas Salk was unable to make progress in his laboratory work on a polio vaccine and to help ease his frustration took a sabbatical to the town of Assisi in Italy; inspired by the light and beauty of the place, he solved his problem, returned to his lab, and created the vaccine. For a detailed discussion of the life and work of Asclepius, see Emma J. Edelstein and Ludwig Edelstein, *Asclepius: Collection and Interpretation of the Testimonies* (Baltimore, MD: Johns Hopkins University Press, 1945).

6. Nancy Gerlach-Spriggs, Richard Enoch Kaufman, and Sam Bass Warner Jr., *Restorative Gardens: The Healing Landscape* (New Haven, CT: Yale University Press, 1998).

7. See Sternberg, *Healing Spaces*, for a discussion of Roger Ulrich's 1984 research documenting that general hospital patients whose beds were located next to windows with a view of a small grove of trees had shorter hospital stays and required fewer doses of pain medication than those with a view of a brick wall.

8. See Gary E. Cordingley, *Stories of Medicine in Athens County, Ohio* (Baltimore, MD: Gateway Press, 2006), 355.

Chapter 1: The Moral Treatment Experiment

1. See James Perry, *Touched with Fire: Five Presidents and the Civil War Battles That Made Them* (New York: Public Affairs, 2003).

2. George W. Paulson and Marion Sherman, *Hilltop: A Hospital and a Sanctuary for Healing; Its Past and Its Future* (Fremont, OH: Lesher, 2008) details the history of the Columbus Asylum for the Insane, originally known as the Ohio Lunatic Asylum.

3. George Knepper, *Ohio and Its People* (Kent, OH: Kent State University, 1989).

4. Thomas Hoover, *The History of Ohio University* (Athens: Ohio University Press, 1954).

5. William Parker Johnson to Julia Blackstone Johnson, June 1, 1861, William Parker Johnson Letters (hereafter cited as Johnson Letters), Manuscript Collection #173, Mahn Center for Archives and Special Collections, Ohio University Libraries.

6. Ibid., January 12, 1862, Johnson Letters.

7. Ibid., July 29, 1862, Johnson Letters.

8. Ibid., January 17, 1863, Johnson Letters.

9. *Hockhocking* is from a Delaware Indian word meaning "bottle," referring to the shape of the river near its origin in central Ohio. James Murphy, *An Archeological History of the Hocking Valley* (Athens: Ohio University Press, 1989). The name of the river was shortened over time to Hocking.

10. "Laying the Cornerstone of the New Asylum: Vast Concourses of People," *Athens (OH) Messenger*, November 12, 1868. The Masonic cornerstone ceremony involved speaking parts from Masonic officials and presentations of corn, wine, and oil. The stone was lowered into its place by mechanical means and declared "well formed, true and trusty." See S. Brent Morris, *Cornerstones of Freemasonry: A Masonic Tradition* (Washington, DC: Masonic Supreme Council, 1993).

11. Nancy Tomes, *The Art of Asylum-Keeping: Thomas Story Kirkbride and the Origins of American Psychiatry* (Philadelphia: University of Pennsylvania Press, 1984). Kirkbride was superintendent of the Pennsylvania Hospital for the Insane from 1840 to 1883.

12. Roy Porter, *Madness: A Brief History* (Oxford: Oxford University Press, 2002), 103–5.

13. William H. Holden, "Sixth Annual Report of the Athens Asylum for the Insane," in *Ohio Executive Documents: Annual Reports for 1879* (Columbus, OH: Nevins and Myers, 1880), 485.

14. Thomas Story Kirkbride, *On the Construction, Organization and General Arrangements of Hospitals for the Insane*, 2nd ed. (1880; repr., New York: Arno Press, 1973). The second edition, published in 1880, revised and expanded the original treatise, published in 1854. Much of the second edition of this treatise can be found online at http://www.kirkbridebuildings.com/about/cogahi/.

15. See www.kirkbridebuildings.com.

16. Kirkbride, *On the Construction* (1880 ed.), 38.

17. Ibid, 59.

18. Personal communication from Pam Callahan, university architect (retired), Ohio University, 2001.

19. Kirkbride, *On the Construction* (1880 ed.), 65.

20. See F. David Roberts, *The Social Conscience of the Early Victorians* (Stanford: Stanford University Press, 2002).

21. See Robert Putnam's analyses of community in America, especially *Bowling Alone: The Collapse and Revival of American Community* (New York: Simon and Schuster, 2001). See also Samuel P. Hayes, *The Response to Industrialism* (Chicago: University of Chicago Press, 1995).

22. Andrew Scull, *The Insanity of Place/The Place of Insanity: Essays on the History of Psychiatry* (New York: Routledge, 2006). See also Michel Foucault, *Madness and Civilization* (New York: Random House, 1965); and Gerald N. Grob, *The Mad among Us: A History of the Care of America's Mentally Ill* (New York: Free Press, 1994). Roy Porter notes, "The asylum solution should be viewed less in terms of central policy than as the site of myriad negotiations of wants, rights, and responsibilities, between diverse parties in a mixed consumer economy with a burgeoning service sector. The confinement (and subsequent release) of a sufferer was commonly less a matter of official fiat than the product of complex bargaining between families, communities, local officials, magistrates, and the superintendents themselves. The initiative to confine might come from varied sources; asylums were used by families no less than by the state; and the law could serve many interests." Porter, *Madness*, 98–99.

23. Rutherford B. Hayes, "Annual Message to the General Assembly," in *Ohio Executive Documents: Annual Reports for 1869* (Columbus, OH: Columbus Printing Company, 1870), 11.

24. Diana S. Waite, "History of Construction of the Athens State Hospital," in *Master Plan for Kennedy Museum: Feasibility Study* (Albany, NY: John G. Waite Associates, 1999), 11.

25. Board of Trustees of the Athens Lunatic Asylum, "Annual Report . . . for 1872," in *Ohio Executive Documents: Annual Reports for 1872* (Columbus, OH: Nevins and Myers, 1873), 11.

26. Kirkbride, *On the Construction* (1880 ed.), 50.

27. Female Patient 454, Athens Mental Health Center Patient Records (hereafter cited as AMHC Patient Records), 1874, Athens Lunatic Asylum Manuscript Collection (MS #263), Mahn Center for Archives and Special Collections, Ohio University Libraries.

28. Female Patient 1296, AMHC Patient Records, 1883.

29. Male Patient 35, AMHC Patient Records, 1874.

30. Probate Judge of Washington County to Supt. Clarke, September 13, 1879, Athens State Hospital Superintendents' Correspondence, Athens Lunatic Asylum Manuscript Collection (MS #263), Mahn Center for Archives and Special Collections, Ohio University Libraries.

31. Male Patient 318, AMHC Patient Records, 1874.

32. The Hocking Valley was the birthplace of the United Mine Workers and the site of a bloody and violent coal miners' strike, which in 1884 prompted the governor to send in the state militia to confront the striking miners. Sheriffs were authorized to use military force, a railroad tunnel and bridges were burned, a citizen was killed, and seven mines were set afire, one of which is still burning today. See Robert L. Daniel, *Athens, Ohio: The Village Years* (Athens: Ohio University Press, 1997).

33. Male Patient 1945, AMHC Patient Records, 1887.

34. Robert Frost, *The Poetry of Robert Frost* (New York: Henry Holt and Co., 1969).

35. Thomas L. Young, "Inaugural Message," in *Ohio Executive Documents: Annual Reports for 1876* (Columbus, OH: Nevins and Myers, 1877), 7.

36. "Samuel Whitely, A Tramp," *Athens (OH) Messenger,* January 8, 1880.

37. Male Patient 1675, AMHC Patient Records, 1885.

38. Male Patient 319, AMHC Patient Records, 1874.

39. See Drew Gilpin Faust, *This Republic of Suffering: Death and the American Civil War* (New York: Alfred A. Knopf, 2008).

40. See Eric Dean, *Shook Over Hell: Post-traumatic Stress, Vietnam, and the Civil War* (Cambridge, MA: Harvard University Press, 1997) for a description of the likely psychological consequences for Civil War veterans, which include symptoms now understood to constitute post-traumatic stress disorder.

41. See David Marlow, *Psychological and Psychosocial Consequences of Combat and Deployment* (Washington, DC: National Defense Research Institute, 2001).

42. Edward F. Noyes, "Annual Message to the General Assembly," in *Ohio Executive Documents: Annual Reports for 1873* (Columbus, OH: Nevin and Myers, 1874), 416.

43. Board of Trustees of the Athens Lunatic Asylum, 1872 annual report, 14.

44. Ibid., 14–15.

45. Ohio asylum superintendents were appointed by the governor and asylum trustees. Superintendents and assistant physicians were typically replaced with the changes of political parties in the state capital of Columbus. Dr. A. B. Richardson was so esteemed (and politically astute), however, that he managed to remain in his superintendent's position at Athens for nine years. Eight medical superintendents led the asylum during the moral treatment years, 1872–96. See Table 4.1; and Gary E. Cordingley, *Stories of Medicine in Athens County, Ohio* (Baltimore, MD: Gateway Press, 2006).

46. For a discussion of the use of various types of restraints, see Deborah Marinski, "Unfortunate Minds: Mental Insanity in Ohio, 1883–1909," PhD diss., University of Toledo, 2006.

47. Board of Trustees of the Athens Lunatic Asylum, 1872 annual report, 10–11.

48. Board of Trustees of the Athens Asylum for the Insane, "Annual Report . . . for 1880," in *Ohio Executive Documents: Annual Report for 1880* (Columbus, OH: Nevins and Myers, 1881), 852.

49. Marinski, "Unfortunate Minds," 144–46.

50. Board of State Charities, "Annual Report . . . ," in *Ohio Executive Documents: Annual Reports for 1880* (Columbus, OH: Nevin and Myers, 1881), 34.

51. Board of Trustees of the Athens Asylum for the Insane, "Annual Report . . . for 1879," in *Ohio Executive Documents: Annual Reports for 1879* (Columbus, OH: Nevins and Myers, 1880), 492.

52. Board of Trustees of the Athens Asylum for the Insane, "Annual Report . . . for 1878," in *Ohio Executive Documents: Annual Reports for 1878* (Columbus, OH: Nevins and Myers, 1879), 405.

53. Ibid., 412.

54. Board of Trustees of the Athens Asylum for the Insane, 1879 annual report, 485.

55. Cordingley, *Stories of Medicine.*

56. Board of Trustees of the Athens Asylum for the Insane, "Annual Report . . . for 1886," in *Ohio Executive Documents: Annual Reports for 1886* (Columbus, OH: Westbote Co., 1887), 44.

Chapter 2: Patients

1. Dr. Lash, an Athens physician, had a dual relationship with the asylum. As a medical witness for patients, he committed them; he was also an asylum trustee in 1876 and 1887–91 and served as board president in 1889.

2. Ohio's commitment documents required community physicians serving as medical witnesses to certify whether patients had epilepsy. Sometimes a physician wrote that a prospective patient had seizures but not epilepsy, perhaps in the hope of improving his or her chances for admission to the asylum.

3. Board of Trustees of the Athens Hospital for the Insane, "Annual Report . . . for 1877," in *Ohio Executive Documents: Annual Reports for 1877* (Columbus, OH: Nevins and Myers, 1878), 412.

4. Board of Trustees of the Athens Asylum for the Insane, "Annual Report . . . for 1879," in *Ohio Executive Documents: Annual Reports for 1879* (Columbus, OH: Nevins and Myers, 1880), 482. In 1893, the Ohio Hospital for Epileptics, the first epilepsy colony in America, opened in the Ohio River town of Gallipolis forty miles from Athens. Housing more than one thousand patients, the hospital facilities included a schoolhouse and a pathology lab, in which was conducted some of the early groundbreaking research into epilepsy. The Athens Lunatic Asylum's Superintendent H. C. Rutter was the founding superintendent of the hospital. He died of poison at the age of sixty-one in Columbus, Ohio. His death was believed to have been suicide. See Gary E. Cordingley, *Stories of Medicine in Athens County, Ohio* (Baltimore, MD: Gateway Press, 2006).

5. Female Patient 1, AMHC Patient Records, 1874.

6. Female Patient 1, *Case Book for Female Patients 1–167,* Athens State Hospital, 1874, State Archives Series 141, Ohio Historical Society Archives/Library.

7. The documents for patients committed by a probate court and admitted by the asylum are held in Athens, Ohio, by Ohio University's Alden Library in the Mahn Center for Archives and Special Collections. Access to these medical records is by permission of the Ohio Department of Mental Health. Documents for thousands of patients are shelved in boxes, beginning in 1874 and running through the early twentieth century.

8. During the asylum's moral treatment years (1874–93), 4,511 persons were admitted or readmitted, for a total of 5,419 admission/readmission processes. Of those, 908 were readmissions. There were 3,556 discharges: of these, 1,883 were considered "recovered," 583 "relieved," 1,085 "unimproved," and 5 "not insane."

9. Board of Trustees of the Athens Hospital for the Insane, "Annual Report . . . for 1876," in *Ohio Executive Documents: Annual Reports for 1876* (Columbus, OH: Nevins and Myers, 1877), 703–4.

10. Wrote the editor of the *Athens Journal* on February 2, 1893, "Athens County roads are now about three feet deep with mud." Robert L. Daniel notes in *Athens, Ohio: The Village Years* (Athens: Ohio University Press, 1997) that citizens were required to perform two days' service on road repair each year or pay three dollars to the county government for maintenance. This service was often neglected, and

roads were in poor condition from mud, ruts, and insufficient drainage. Superintendent A. B. Richardson in his 1888 report to the board of trustees described the condition of local roads as "wretched."

11. Pinel's was a taxonomy of four kinds of mental illness, all of which correspond to twenty-first-century diagnostic categories: melancholia, which included depression and anxiety; mania with delirium, which corresponded approximately with bipolar disorder; mania without delirium, which included mania; and dementia, which was an umbrella term for forgetfulness and memory loss, loss of judgment, continuous activity, and diminished reactions/perception of external stimuli. See Philippe Pinel, *Traité médico-philosophique sur l'aliénation mentale*, trans. as *A Treatise on Insanity* by D. D. Davis (1806; Birmingham, AL: Classics of Medicine Library, 1983).

12. For example, medical witness Dr. H. M. Lash noted that the insanity of one female patient (described as a single resident of rural southeastern Ohio, age twenty-one, of moderate education) was caused by walking in a creek while menstruating: "She was doing kitchen work in Athens, went into the Country on a visit to relations on Saturday, she was menstruating at the time, took off her shoes and walked in the creek." Female Patient 2, AMHC Patient Records, 1874.

13. American physicians sometimes used the nineteenth-century French term *onanisme* for masturbation.

14. The dynamometer measured the strength of the grip of the hand.

15. Male Patient 1, *Case Book for Male Patients 1–179*, Athens State Hospital, 1874, State Archives Series 141, Ohio Historical Society Archives/Library. The handwritten commitment notes, case notes, and letters serving as primary research material for this book contain spelling errors and variants, as well as capitalizations that may be unfamiliar to the twenty-first-century reader. These are reproduced in the text just as they were written by the physicians, probate judges, patients, and family members.

16. Male Patient 221, AMHC Patient Records, 1874.

17. Male Patient 334, AMHC Patient Records, 1874.

18. Male Patient 47, AMHC Patient Records, 1874. Also Male Patient 47, *Case Book for Male Patients 1–179*.

19. Suicide, and perhaps mental illness, was not a stranger to this patient's family. His brother had hanged himself after returning home from Longview Asylum in Cincinnati.

20. Male Patient 30, AMHC Patient Records, 1874. Also Male Patient 30, *Case Book for Male Patients 1–179*.

21. Nineteenth-century Ohio, like many other states, had a system of county homes for persons who had no means of support. Established as a less expensive means than providing cash allowances, the homes, also called infirmaries, provided a permanent place of residence for individuals and families. See www.poorhousestory.com/history.

22. Unless otherwise specified, the information for all of these patients can be found in the AMHC Patient Records, organized by each patient's number.

23. This quotation is from *Case Book for Female Patients 1–167*.

24. A drummer and historian of his regiment, the husband served between 1861 and 1865 at the siege of Corinth, Chickamauga, the siege of Atlanta, and the battle of Jonesboro, among others.

25. Puerperal infection is a bacterial infection following childbirth.

26. Female Patient 377, AMHC Patient Records, 1874.

27. P. Ricord, *A Practical Treatise on Venereal Diseases* (New York: Gordon, 1842). Available online at http://pds.lib.harvard.edu/pds/view/6560410?n=11&imagesize=1200&jp2Res=.25.

28. The state of West Virginia was formed in 1863, and in 1874 some in Ohio, perhaps out of habit, still referred to the land south and east of the Ohio River as Virginia.

29. The patient's family history contained suicide: her paternal grandmother, two paternal uncles, a paternal aunt, and a paternal cousin all hanged themselves.

30. Male Patient 819, letters to his family, undated, Athens State Hospital Superintendents' Correspondence.

31. The Victorian asylum term for *escaping* was *eloping,* and both men and women eloped from the asylum, though men eloped in greater numbers. In 1884, for example, Dr. A. B. Richardson's annual report to the trustees noted seventeen successful elopements: fourteen males and three females. The annual budget of the Athens asylum included funds, essentially a bounty, paid to townsmen to retrieve patients. April brought the greatest expense in retrieving patients, perhaps because the coming of spring's warm weather after the long Ohio River valley winter encouraged patients to leave.

32. Settled in 1788 by the Ohio Company of Associates in the Northwest Territory, Marietta was named for Queen Marie Antoinette of France to honor France for its help in the American Revolution. Located along the trade route of the Ohio River, Marietta grew into a mercantile center known for ship-building and trade based on the many apple orchards in the area. The Marquis de Lafayette visited Marietta in 1825.

33. Capt. Ben F. Hall to Superintendent W. H. Holden, July 8, 1880, Athens State Hospital Superintendents' Correspondence.

34. Male Patient 1060 to John Smart, undated, Athens State Hospital Superintendents' Correspondence.

35. Male Patient 176, *Case Book for Male Patients 1–179.* The asylum's annual liquor budget ranged anywhere from $303.34 to $3,843.23 and included ale, bourbon, rye whiskey, wine, gin, port, and sherry.

36. Male Patient 1663, AMHC Patient Records, 1874.

37. Male Patient 171, AMHC Patient Records, 1874.

38. Male Patient 41, *Case Book for Male Patients 1–179.*

39. Female Patient 28, AMHC Patient Records, 1874.

40. Male Patient 209, AMHC Patient Records, 1874.

41. Male Patient 1921, AMHC Patient Records, 1887.

42. Female Patient 17, *Case Book for Female Patients 1–167.*

43. Male Patient 12, *Case Book for Male Patients, 1–179.*

44. The oldest of the three cemeteries, where nineteenth-century patients are buried, lies just above the hospital on a site carved into a hillside. The headstones are numbered rather than named, except for the few erected by friends or family. Two other cemeteries lie a quarter mile or more from the main asylum building and contain the graves of patients up through the 1970s. All are owned by the Ohio Department of Mental Health and are tended by a volunteer cemetery committee, part of the Athens Chapter of NAMI (National Alliance on Mental Illness) and headed by Dr. Thomas Walker of Ohio University.

45. Female Patient 49, *Case Book for Female Patients 1–167.*

46. Female Patient 49, AMHC Patient Records, 1874.

47. By 1874, Athens was connected by rail with Columbus to the north, Parkersburg (West Virginia) to the east, and Cincinnati to the west. The town was served by the B&O Short Line, the Hocking Valley Railroad, and the Marietta and Cincinnati railroad. Daniel, *Athens, Ohio,* 220–25.

48. Male Patient 38, *Case Book for Male Patients 1–179.*

49. Female Patient 13, *Case Book for Female Patients 1–167.*

50. Female Patient 26, *Case Book for Female Patients 1–167.*

51. Holden, "Sixth Annual Report," 481.

52. Board of Trustees of the Athens Asylum for the Insane, "Annual Report . . . for 1887," in *Ohio Executive Documents: Annual Reports for 1887* (Columbus, OH: Westbote Co., 1888), 237.

53. Board of Trustees of the Athens Asylum for the Insane, 1880 annual report, 851–52.

54. Female Patient 1509, AMHC Patient Records, 1874.

55. The case files of the asylum at Athens list several dozen persons in the nineteenth century who were turned away because asylum physicians determined that they were not mentally ill. AMHC Patient Records, 1874–93.

56. Derek H. Alderman, "Integrating Space into a Reactive Theory of the Asylum: Evidence from Post–Civil War Georgia," *Health and Place* 3 (1997): 111–22. Alderman studied admissions to Georgia's state insane asylum during the post–Civil War Reconstruction period. He argues for a re-active theory of asylums, in which the shifting needs of families and communities determine who is hospitalized. Greater social distance—less closely knit families and communities—increased family and community needs for an institution to provide care.

57. Her case history reads, "About 6 or 7 years ago during menstruation she was going to some night meetings; in crossing a run flowing with ice, she fell off her horse into the run, went on to the meeting and remained in that condition all evening. Since, she has periodically spasm or convul-sions, but not amounting to epilepsy. . . . Medical treatment has been I believe entirely wanting, except what treatment she may have received in the Lunatic Asylum at Dayton."

58. Female Patient 52, AMHC Patient Records, 1874.

59. Before 1874, the nearest state hospitals for the insane were in Cincinnati in southwestern Ohio and Columbus in the center of the state. No doubt the Athens asylum was a more attractive option for families in southeastern Ohio. See Alderman, "Integrating Space."

60. Female Patient 377, AMHC Patient Records, 1874.

61. The father's physician noted on the medical certificate that "his mind has been somewhat impared for two years but he has become much worse since his son became insane. Duration about two years. Cause: probably difficulty with neighbors resulting in law suits. The said patient has made attempts of violence upon others."

62. The files of the asylum's Superintendents' Correspondence contain letters to family at home written by patients and never mailed, letters from family members inquiring about the status of patients, and letters written to patients by family members. Male Patient 706 left a set of letters written three years after he was hospitalized. Never mailed, his letters were retained in a file among the papers of the medical superintendent.

63. Male Patient 706 to his family, June 27, 1880, Athens State Hospital Superintendents' Correspondence.

64. Male Patient 706 to his family, August 31, 1880, ibid. The salutations and dates of letters by Male Patient 706 were intricate. For example:

> Tuesday P.M. August 31th U. S. Olympic Period A. D. 1880. Lunar Callendar. Mean and True Time. Dear Son and Daughter. I Address your Letter at Hamilton County State of Ohio. Wishing you much Joy in your "New Departure" in Life's chequered Journey. But I must go back to another Age! Another Epoch! When you the Genus Homo Pater Familias: The Heirsute Knight! Was Living with your Eldest Brother at the Center of the suspension Bridge across La Belle Riviere!!
>
> And I will tell you that this is Wednesday Morning the first day of September and has been since midnight. That the sun rose here this morning! At five hours! Twenty eight Minutes. A.M. Cancer or Crab Fish Constellation five Days. South's nine Hours. Thirty six minutes! Aspects of Planets . . . Uranus! And the sun . . . Circumcision High Tides. Four Hours. Four Minutes. A.M. Four Hours given Four Minutes! P.M. Egyptian Jewish Calendar Collendar. 5640 January 14th Rosh: Hashana: Shebat. December 28th! Rosh! Shanah! Period. The creation of the world the age of Lucifer: Pluto, Beelzebub Satan's. And the 14th of April A. D. 1842 and the 8th Day of October 1843! Your own birthdays! And my own Age: Pliny, Bulwen Chateaubria. By Rousseau, Napoleon Bonapart. (Ibid.)

65. Ibid., August 30, 1880.

66. A reference to the presidential election of 1876, in which Samuel Tilden won the popular vote and Ohioan Rutherford B. Hayes won the electoral vote. For a detailed discussion, see Paul Leland Haworth, *The Hayes-Tilden Disputed Presidential Election of 1876* (Cleveland: Burrows, 1906).

67. Male Patient 706 to his family, August 31, 1880, Athens State Hospital Superintendents' Correspondence.

68. Alderman, "Integrating Space." Alderman analyzed commitment data to the state asylum in post–Civil War Georgia and found that families' willingness to commit a family member was related to the spatial distance to the institution: families who lived close by were more willing to seek commitment than those living farther away.

69. Male Patient 9, *Case Book for Male Patients 1–179.*

Chapter 3: Architecture

1. Joseph T. Hannibal and Richard A. Davis, "The Cleves Tunnel, a Rare Extant Example of the Use of Buena Vista Stone for a Canal Structure near Cincinnati, Ohio," in *Proceedings of the 40th Forum on the Geology of Industrial Minerals,* ed. N. R. Shafer and D. A. DeChurch, 64–69, Indiana Geological Survey Occasional Paper 67 (Bloomington: Indiana Geological Survey, 2004). Buena Vista freestone, sometimes called sandstone, is actually a siltstone, which is finer grained than sandstone. It is called "freestone" because it can be cut in any direction. The freestone for the asylum likely came from quarries near the town of Buena Vista in southern Ohio.

2. Board of Trustees of the Athens Lunatic Asylum, 1872 annual report, 14.

3. Steven D. Blankenbeker, "The Paving Brick Industry in Ohio," *Ohio Geology* 3 (1999): 1.

4. Interview with Pam Callahan, architect, Ohio University (retired), November 5, 2010.

5. New Advertisements, *Athens (OH) Messenger,* February 11, 1868.

6. Diana S. Waite, "History of Construction of the Athens State Hospital," in *Master Plan for Kennedy Museum: Feasibility Study* (Albany: John G. Waite Associates, 1999), 3–17.

7. Robert L. Daniel, *Athens, Ohio: The Village Years* (Athens: Ohio University Press, 1997).

8. Thomas Story Kirkbride, *On the Construction, Organization and General Arrangements of Hospitals for the Insane, with some Remarks on Insanity and Its Treatment* (Philadelphia: Pennsylvania Hospital for the Insane, 1854). The second edition of 1880 is available in part online at http://www .kirkbridebuildings.com/about/cogahi/.

9. Henry Wotton, *The Elements of Architecture by Sir Henry Wotton, a Facsimili Reprint of the First Edition (London, 1624),* ed. Frederick Hard (Charlottesville: University Press of Virginia, 1968), lxix. Wotton's elements of well-building are derived from the Vetruvian source: *firmitatis, utilitatis, venustatis.*

10. Board of Trustees of the Athens Lunatic Asylum, 1872 annual report, 15.

11. Board of Trustees of the Athens Lunatic Asylum, 1872 annual report, 3–16.

12. George W. Paulson and Marion E. Sherman, *Hilltop: A Hospital and a Sanctuary for Healing, Its Past and Its Future* (Fremont, OH: Lesher Printers, 2008), 59–60. The building caught fire on a November evening; the Columbus fire department safely removed 314 patients, who were then housed in private homes and at the Ohio Deaf and Dumb Asylum. Six patients suffocated.

13. Board of Trustees of the Athens Lunatic Asylum, 1872 annual report, 10–11.

14. *A History of Cleveland and Its Environs* (Chicago: Lewis Publishing, 1918).

15. Waite, "History of Construction."

16. Ibid.

17. Board of Trustees of the Athens Lunatic Asylum, 1872 annual report, 5.

18. Board of Trustees of the Athens Lunatic Asylum, 1872 annual report, 15.

19. Gerald N. Grob, *The Mad among Us: A History of the Care of America's Mentally Ill* (New York: Free Press, 1994), 66.

20. Board of Trustees of the Athens Lunatic Asylum, 1872 annual report, 12–13.

21. Board of Trustees of the Athens Asylum for the Insane, 1880 annual report, 855.

22. Grob, *Mad among Us,* 66.

23. Andrew Scull, *Social Order/Mental Disorder: Anglo-American Psychiatry in Historical Perspective* (Berkeley: University of California Press, 1989), 225–26.

24. Board of Trustees of the Athens Lunatic Asylum, 1872 annual report, 12.

25. Kirkbride, *On the Construction* (1854 ed.), 24.

26. Board of Trustees of the Athens Lunatic Asylum, 1872 annual report, 13.

27. Ibid., 14.

28. Board of Trustees of the Athens Asylum for the Insane, "Annual Report . . . for 1893," in *Ohio Executive Documents: Annual Reports for 1893* (Columbus, OH: Laning Printing Co., 1894), 629.

29. Board of Trustees of the Athens Asylum for the Insane, 1880 annual report, 854–56.

Chapter 4: Politics

1. The Ohio legislature appropriated $621,000 in 1868 for the construction of the Athens Lunatic Asylum. Depending on the conversion method used to compute the relative value, that amount could equate to anywhere from about $9 million to more than $1 billion in today's currency (see, for instance, the computations in the relative values calculators at www.MeasuringWorth.com).

2. Called the Long Depression by economic historians, the depression of the years 1873–79 was precipitated by the Panic of 1873 and the failure of the Philadelphia banking concern of Jay Cooke on September 18, 1873.

3. Board of State Charities, "Annual Report," in *Ohio Executive Documents: Annual Reports for 1879* (Columbus, OH: Nevins and Myers, 1880), 563–92.

4. Gerald N. Grob, *The Mad among Us: A History of the Care of America's Mentally Ill* (New York: Free Press, 1994), 23–53. Although the early Southern asylums were established with a nod toward moral treatment philosophy, they were mostly custodial. The motivation for their founding was for the most part protecting community and family from behaviors exhibited by individuals with mental illness considered intrusive or dangerous.

5. Nancy Tomes, *The Art of Asylum-Keeping: Thomas Story Kirkbride and the Origins of American Psychiatry* (Philadelphia: University of Pennsylvania Press, 1994), 6.

6. Grob, *Mad among Us*, 46.

7. David Gollaher, *Voice for the Mad: The Life of Dorothea Dix* (New York: Free Press, 1995).

8. Ibid., 395–422.

9. Frank B. Norbury, "Dorothea Dix and the Founding of Illinois' First Mental Hospital," *Journal of the Illinois State Historical Society* 92 (1999): 13–29.

10. Deborah Marinski, "Unfortunate Minds: Mental Insanity in Ohio 1883–1909" (PhD diss., University of Toledo, 2006).

11. Thomas Hoover, *The History of Ohio University* (Athens: Ohio University Press, 1954), 123–26.

12. Katherine Ziff, David Thomas, and Patricia Beamish, "Asylum and Community: The Athens Lunatic Asylum in Nineteenth-Century Ohio," *History of Psychiatry* 19 (2008): 409–32.

13. Katherine Ziff, "Asylum and Community: Connections between the Athens Lunatic Asylum and the Village of Athens, 1867–1893," PhD diss., Ohio University, 2004.

14. Board of State Charities, 1880 annual report, 24.

15. Ibid., 38.

16. Rutherford B. Hayes, August 8, 1875, in *The Diary and Letters of Rutherford B. Hayes, Nineteenth President of the United States*, ed. Charles Richard Williams, 3:289 (Columbus: Ohio State Archeological and Historical Society, 1922). http://www.ohiohistory.org/onlinedoc/hayes/index.cfm.

17. Ibid., April 6, 1876, 3:311.

18. Ibid., April 24, 1891, 4:647.

19. Ibid., December 1854, 1:473. Russell H. Conwell, in *Life and Service of Governor Rutherford B. Hayes* (Boston: Franklin Press, 1876), refers to the defendant as Nancy Farrar, the "idiotic poisoner" (62).

20. Hayes, January 25, 1873, *Diary and Letters*, 3: 146.

21. Ibid., 227. Dr. Webb died a few years later. Hayes wrote that Webb had been "out of health" several years and his superintendency of Longview had left him unwell: "The location was a bad

one being near the canal. Chills and fever prevailed. Doctor Webb was never rid of chills and fever after he left Longview. In addition to this he had severe headaches. He was of a bilious temperament and quite corpulent. His sudden death was therefore not a surprise to us." Hayes feared at times for Webb's mental health: "He occasionally had melancholy spells . . . after the failure of his health the morbid tendency of his nature became strong. . . . I sometimes feared that he would become insane. There were occasional symptoms of it. He distrusted at times his nearest friends. Dr. Comegys, a friend and connection, feared that he might glide into insanity." Hayes, April 28, 1880, *Diary and Letters,* 3:597.

22. Ibid., June 12, 1873, *Diary and Letters,* 3:244.

23. Gary E. Cordingley, *Stories of Medicine in Athens County, Ohio* (Baltimore, MD: Gateway Press, 2006). 3–4.

24. Board of Trustees of the Athens Asylum for the Insane, 1877 annual report.

25. Board of State Charities, 1880 annual report.

26. Cordingley, *Stories of Medicine,* 313–15.

27. John Friday to Phillip Zenner, April 22, 1879, Dr. Phillip Zenner Collection (MS #44), Mahn Center for Archives and Special Collections, Ohio University Libraries. John Friday was the son-in-law and partner of Samuel Zenner in the family business D. Zenner and Sons, an Athens clothing establishment. The Zenners furnished the asylum with dry goods, notions, and lengths of fabric.

28. John Friday to Phillip Zenner, June 9, 1879, ibid.

29. Henry Zenner to Phillip Zenner, April 1879, ibid.

30. David Zenner to Phillip Zenner, April 29, 1879, ibid.

31. Board of Trustees of the Athens Asylum for the Insane, 1879 annual report, 486–91.

32. Ziff, "Asylum and Community" (2004), 110.

33. Board of State Charities, 1879 annual report, 582–83.

34. Local Matters, *Athens (OH) Messenger,* January 29, 1880.

35. Board of State Charities, 1880 annual report, 594.

36. Board of Trustees of the Athens Asylum for the Insane, 1879 annual report.

37. Local Matters, *Athens (OH) Messenger,* May 27, 1880.

38. Male Patient 922 to a Friend, 1880, Athens State Hospital Superintendents' Correspondence.

39. Local Matters, *Athens (OH) Messenger,* May 27, 1880.

40. Hazel Phillips and Lawrence Gray, *Governors of Ohio* (Columbus: Ohio Historical Society, 1952).

41. The annual operating budget in 1890, for example, was $110,000. Using a consumer price index estimate (www.measuringworth.com), this converts to approximately $2.7 million at 2010 value.

42. Board of Trustees of the Athens Asylum for the Insane, "Annual Report . . . for 1889," in *Ohio Executive Documents: Annual Reports for 1889* (Columbus, OH: Westbote Co., 1890), 1164.

43. Board of Trustees of the Athens Asylum for the Insane, 1893 annual report, 617–25.

44. Alienists, the name by which nineteenth-century asylum superintendents were known, because their patients were persons who had been alienated by family and society, organized in 1844 to form the Association of Medical Superintendents of American Institutions for the Insane (AMSAII), which in the twentieth century became the American Psychiatric Association. Roy Porter, *Madness: A Brief History* (Oxford: Oxford University Press, 2002), 153–54.

45. http://www.nlm.nih.gov/hmd/medtour/elizabeths.html.

46. Memorial by Dr. Henly Rutter, in Proceedings of the American Medico-Psychological Association at the Sixtieth Annual Meeting, held in St. Louis, Missouri, May 30–June 3, 1904 (published by the American Medico-Psychological Association in 1904, downloaded from Google digitized documents August 4, 2009). Other memorials were written by Henry C. Eyman, superintendent of Massillon State Hospital in Ohio, and William Henry Scott, third president of Ohio State University in Columbus, Ohio, and professor at Ohio University, 1869–72.

Chapter 5: Landscape

1. Board of Trustees of the Athens Lunatic Asylum, 1872 annual report, 11.

2. The construction and alteration of the landscape must have made a deep impression upon Ballard, as he wrote again in the summer: "The work on the Assylum [*sic*] is progressing with great rapidity. It will look splendidly from various points in our town. The forest the other side of the river is all cut down." John Ballard to his son, August 10, 1869, Ballard Collection, MS #23, Mahn Center for Archives and Special Collections, Ohio University Libraries.

3. Board of Trustees of the Athens Asylum for the Insane, 1880 annual report.

4. For a discussion of Olmsted's work and life, see Witold Rybczynski, *A Clearing in the Distance* (New York: Scribner, 1999).

5. Herman Haerlin's floral show filled a large exhibition hall still used today for the same purpose at the Ohio State Fair in Columbus, "gaily decorated with an incredible botanical display." The display was in the style of today's flower show competitions in which tableaux are created by individuals seeking prizes. Haerlin's exhibition featured a combination of his horticultural artistry—cherry trees filled with orchids and lawns with beds of flowers—plus individual entries of scenes created with palms, ferns, roses, "rustic stands and fine rustic work," tuberoses, pomegranates, coleus, fuchsias, grasses, succulents, and a miniature garden with fountains. Prizes were awarded for floral design, cut flowers, and bouquets. Haerlin's exhibition hall attracted "large crowds of visitors, highly enjoyed by the public." Herman Haerlin, "Report of Commissioner Haerlin," in *Annual Report of the Ohio State Board of Agriculture for 1888*, 58–59 (Columbus, OH: Westbote Co., 1881). Available online through Google.

6. Board of Trustees of the Athens Hospital for the Insane, 1876 annual report.

7. Ibid., 715–16.

8. Ibid.

9. Board of Trustees of the Athens Hospital for the Insane, 1877 annual report, 413.

10. Ibid., 417.

11. Board of Trustees of the Athens Asylum for the Insane, 1878 annual report, 408–409.

12. His name, spelled Linck in the 1880 census, was likely "Americanized" to Link.

13. "Grounds of State Hospital Most Beautiful of Middle West," *Athens (OH) Messenger*, May 3, 1955.

14. "Death of George Link, Landscape Gardener at Hospital for Thirty-two Years," *Athens (OH) Messenger*, August 16, 1903.

15. The asylum payroll referred to him according to the work for which he was hired, but most often grading foreman was his function. Payroll records also referred to him as fireman, fencing foreman, florist, gardener, and grade boss.

16. Board of Trustees of the Athens Hospital for the Insane, 1877 annual report, 413–14.

17. Board of Trustees of the Athens Asylum for the Insane, "Annual Report . . . for 1885," in *Ohio Executive Documents: Annual Reports for 1885* (Columbus, OH: Westbote Co., 1886), 984.

18. Board of Trustees of the Athens Hospital for the Insane, 1876 annual report, 716–17.

19. Board of Trustees of the Athens Asylum for the Insane, "Annual Report . . . for 1881," in *Ohio Executive Documents: Annual Reports for 1881* (Columbus, OH: G. J. Brand and Co., 1882), 9.

20. Board of Trustees of the Athens Asylum for the Insane, "Annual Report . . . for 1883," in *Ohio Executive Documents: Annual Reports for 1883* (Columbus, OH: G. J. Brand and Co., 1884), 634.

21. In *Souder v. Brennan* (1973), the court ruled that patient-workers in a mental hospital are "employees" covered by the provisions of the Fair Labor Standards Act and must be paid for their work.

22. Board of Trustees of the Athens Asylum for the Insane, 1883 annual report, 634.

23. Board of Trustees of the Athens Hospital for the Insane, 1876 annual report, 715.

24. Ibid.

25. Board of Trustees of the Athens Hospital for the Insane, 1877 annual report, 716.

26. Board of Trustees of the Athens Asylum for the Insane, 1885 annual report.

27. Ibid.

28. Board of Trustees of the Athens Asylum for the Insane, 1893 annual report.

29. The asylum's airing courts, fully enclosed courtyards, were originally featured as safe places for outdoor exercise. However, Dr. Richardson, a leader in the American asylum antirestraint movement, considered walled exercise courtyards a method of restraint and advocated their abandonment. Dr. Richardson wrote a lengthy rationale for this change in a report to the governor: "As ordinarily employed I do not think these are productive of much good. On the contrary, they are very liable to do harm. The attendant is strongly tempted to let the high walls take the place of his own vigilance, and gradually forms habits of indolence and carelessness, which soon extend to his duties indoors as well as affect those outside. The patients thus left to themselves are permitted to destroy shrubbery and clothing, to become quarrelsome with each other, and to contract habits of uncleanliness and immorality." Writing from his experience as superintendent at Athens and other asylums, Richardson explained, "The humiliation of the confinement by high walls has also an undoubted moral effect. I have seen these enclosures become perfect bedlams in their confusion, and the profanity and obscenity in language and conduct was certainly not without a shock, even to persons accustomed to the remarkable exhibitions in that direction among the violent insane. It is no wonder that patients frequently prefer to remain in the ward rather than to enjoy the fresh air and sunlight of heaven under such unpleasant and humiliating surroundings. And I have in my own experience frequently seen the same patient, who kept in the ward or confined to the walled enclosure, was continually planning escapes or discontentedly demanding release, come in from an afternoon spent in a long stroll over the hills for miles in the country, contented and quiet and enjoy food and bed. . . . [W]here institutions are in a city they may sometimes be a necessity, but in our case [we] have found the instances demanding their use to be extremely rare." Both quotations from Board of Trustees of the Athens Asylum for the Insane, 1882 annual report, 823.

30. Board of Trustees of the Athens Asylum for the Insane, 1883 annual report, 633.

31. Board of Trustees of the Athens Asylum for the Insane, 1882 annual report, 823–24.

32. Board of Trustees of the Athens Asylum for the Insane, 1879 annual report, 487.

33. Board of Trustees of the Athens Asylum for the Insane, 1878 annual report, 412.

34. S. C. Tipton, *Athens County Illustrated Progress of One Hundred Years Centennial* (Athens, OH: Messenger and Herald, 1897), 12.

35. Male Patient 8, AMHC Patient Records, 1874.

36. Board of Trustees of the Athens Asylum for the Insane, 1878 annual report, 411–12.

37. Board of Trustees of the Athens Asylum for the Insane, 1879 annual report, 488.

38. Board of Trustees of the Athens Asylum for the Insane, 1881 annual report, 9.

39. Board of Trustees of the Athens Asylum for the Insane, 1883 annual report, 732.

40. Board of Trustees of the Athens Asylum for the Insane, 1886 annual report, 39–40.

41. "History of Athens Mental Health Center: Hospital-Community Relationship Spans 121 Years," *Athens (OH) Messenger*, March 21, 1988.

Chapter 6: Caregivers

1. The asylum's resident officers were the superintendent and his wife the matron, assistant physicians, steward, and storekeeper.

2. Attendant Supervisor to Dr. Rutter, 1878, Athens State Hospital Superintendents' Correspondence.

3. Board of Trustees of the Athens Asylum for the Insane, 1886 annual report.

4. Nancy Theriot, "Diagnosing Unnatural Motherhood: Nineteenth Century Physicians and Puerperal Insanity," in *Women and Health in America: Historical Readings,* ed. Judith Walzer Leavitt (Madison: University of Wisconsin Press, 1999), 403–17.

5. Charles I. Cerney, *The Chronicles of Medicine in Muskingum County, Ohio, 1800–2000* (Zanesville, OH: privately published), 340.

6. Hamblin resigned from the asylum in 1888 as a part of political reorganization; Dr. Richardson left as well. A few years later, Hamblin reappeared on Ohio's state asylum scene when he was appointed steward of the Toledo Insane Asylum by Governor McKinley's administration. Noted the *Athens (OH) Messenger* on January 12, 1893, "Nothing in recent years has so stirred up the republican politicians of the state . . . as the appointment of Mr. Hamblin as the steward of the Toledo Insane Asylum. Mr. Hamblin is a democrat and the republican trustees wisely concluded, after a thorough canvass of the field, that a better man was not available."

7. Katherine Ziff, David Thomas, and Patricia Beamish, "Asylum and Community: The Athens Lunatic Asylum in Nineteenth-Century Ohio," *History of Psychiatry* 19 (2008): 409–32. Athens merchants benefited from asylum purchases. Grocers A. L. Roach and Son, Davis & Son, Hiram Bingham, J. H. Vorhes & Brothers and W. H. Brown & Co. sold the asylum flour, fruit, garden seed, eggs, butter, beans, poultry, coffee, ham, vinegar, apples, oysters, tea, sugar, tobacco, fuses and powder, soap, and cinnamon. C. H. Warden & Brothers sold butter and eggs, sometimes in quantities as great as 339 dozen eggs per month. The steward purchased from the Athens Water-Wheel and Machine Company steam- and water-supply equipment. Stranathan & Co. sold to the steward items such as forty-eight dozen pairs of underwear, a hogshead of New Orleans sugar, barrels of rice and dried corn, soap, tea, whiskey, undershirts, and 1,500 yards of printed fabric. W. R. Calkins & Brothers sold the steward jelly cake pans, cook pans, and dish pans. He brought from W. H. Potter cigars, fish, kraut, onions, and potatoes. The old establishment of Van Vorhes & Bartlett kept the asylum in coal oil and hardware. D. Zenner & Sons provided dry goods, notions, and lengths of fabric, as did M. Selig & Co.

8. Ibid., 420.

9. Lucinda Pickett to her mother, April 23, 1874, Lucinda Pickett Connett Collection (hereafter cited as Connett Correspondence), Athens County Museum and Historical Society, Athens, Ohio.

10. Gerald Grob, *The Mad among Us: A History of the Care of America's Mentally Ill* (New York: Macmillan, 1994), 92–95.

11. Lucinda Pickett Connett to her mother, March 6, 1876, Connett Correspondence.

12. Board of Trustees of the Athens Asylum for the Insane, "Annual Report for 1888," in *Ohio Executive Documents: Annual Reports for 1888* (Columbus, OH: Westbote Co., 1889), 665.

13. Ibid.

14. Sarah C. Sitton, *Life at the Texas State Lunatic Asylum, 1857–1997* (College Station: Texas A&M University Press, 1999), 74–76.

15. Board of Trustees of the Athens Asylum for the Insane, 1888 annual report, 1162.

16. Henry C. Eyman, "Massillon State Hospital," in *The Institutional Care of the Insane in the United States and Canada*, ed. Henry Mills Hurd et al. (Baltimore, MD: Johns Hopkins University Press, 1916), 3:330–32.

17. Ziff, Thomas, and Beamish, "Asylum and Community," 416.

18. Among other engagements, his unit fought at Perryville, Chickamauga, the Siege of Atlanta, Jonesboro, and the March to Washington. Civil War Soldiers and Sailors System website: http://www.itd.nps.gov/cwss/.

19. Nancy Tomes, *The Art of Asylum-Keeping: Thomas Story Kirkbride and the Origins of American Psychiatry* (Philadelphia: University of Pennsylvania Press, 1994), 199–202.

20. Board of Trustees of the Athens Asylum for the Insane, 1887 annual report, 228–72.

21. John _____ to Dr. Henly Rutter regarding Male Patient 794, September 7, 1880, Athens State Hospital Superintendents' Correspondence.

22. John _____ to his brother, September 7, 1880, ibid.

23. Relative of Male Patient 603 to Superintendent of Asylum, September 1, 1880, ibid.

24. Relative of Male Patient 1064 to Dr. Kelly, August 19, 1880, ibid.

25. Probate Judge B. Stove to Superintendent Holden, February 16, 1879, ibid.

26. W. H. Holden to Supervisor J. H. Carpenter, August 19, 1879, ibid.

27. Granddaughter of Male Patient 152 to Superintendent Henly Rutter, September 21, 1880, ibid.

28. See Grob, *Mad among Us;* Andrew Scull, *Social Order/Mental Disorder: Anglo-American Psychiatry in Historical Perspective* (Berkeley: University of California Press, 1989), 118–61; and Roy Porter, *Madness: A Brief History* (Oxford: Oxford University Press, 2002), 134–55.

Epilogue

1. S. Weir Mitchell, "Address before the Fiftieth Annual Meeting of the American Medico-Psychological Association, Held in Philadelphia, May 16th, 1894," *American Journal of Psychiatry* 151 (1994): 28–36 (reprinted from *The Journal of Nervous and Mental Disease,* July 1894).

2. Gerald Grob notes that "surviving evidence suggests that moral treatment achieved—even by contemporary standards—some striking successes. Although claims about curability rates were undoubtedly exaggerated, there is little doubt that many individuals benefited from hospitalization. In the 1880s the superintendent of the Worcester hospital undertook a follow-up study of over a thousand patients discharged as recovered on their only or last admission . . . data were accumulated on 984 individuals . . . of these nearly 58% of those discharged as recovered had functioned in a community setting without a relapse." Grob, "The Transformation of the Mental Hospital in the United States," *American Behavioral Scientist* 28 (1985): 639–54.

3. Ibid.

4. Nancy Tomes, *The Art of Asylum-Keeping: Thomas Story Kirkbride and the Origins of American Psychiatry* (Philadelphia: University of Pennsylvania Press, 1984), 200.

5. George W. Paulson and Marion E. Sherman note in their history of the Hilltop asylum in Columbus that Pliny Earle, a founder of the American Psychiatric Association, wrote in 1864, "We freely acknowledge that the Ohio State system appears to us to be the best hitherto devised in America." Paulson and Sherman, *Hilltop: A Hospital and a Sanctuary for Healing, Its Past and its Future* (Fremont, OH: Lesher Printers, 2008), 79–80.

6. Ibid.

7. Gerald Grob, *The Mad among Us: A History of the Care of America's Mentally Ill* (New York: Macmillan, 1994), 109–12.

8. Ibid., 135–38.

9. Barbara Floyd et al., *From Institutions to Independence: A History of People with Disabilities in Northwest Ohio—An Exhibition* (Toledo: Ward M. Canaday Center for Special Collections, University Libraries, University of Toledo, 2009).

10. For a detailed account of this incident, as well as many firsthand accounts of life at the Athens asylum in the twentieth century, see Gary E. Cordingley, *Stories of Medicine in Athens County, Ohio* (Baltimore, MD: Gateway Press, 2006).

11. Ibid.

12. News article from the *Athens (OH) Messenger and Herald,* February 15, 1907, quoted in ibid.

13. Annual Report of the Athens State Hospital, Athens, Ohio, 1913, 2. This report, maintained in the superintendents' correspondence files, was typewritten and presumably forwarded to the Ohio Board of Administration.

14. Andrew Scull, "Psychiatry and Social Control in the Nineteenth and Twentieth Centuries," *History of Psychiatry* 2 (1991): 155–56.

15. Andrew Scull, *Social Order/Mental Disorder: Anglo-American Psychiatry in Historical Perspective* (Berkeley: University of California Press, 1989), 68–69.

16. Athens State Hospital, *Thirty-Eighth Report of the Athens State Hospital for the Year Ending November 15, 1913 to the Ohio Board of Administration* (Athens, OH: n.p., 1913).

17. Ibid., 4.

18. Ibid., 5.

19. John H. Berry, "Historical Sketch No. 17: The Athens State Hospital . . . 1929," report prepared for the Ohio Department of Public Welfare, vertical files for the Athens Mental Health Center in Mahn Center for Archives and Special Collections, Ohio University Libraries.

20. J. Fremont Bateman and H. Warren Dunham, "The State Mental Hospital as a Specialized Community Experience," *American Journal of Psychiatry* 105 (1948): 445–48.

21. For an account of the life and work of Dr. Freeman, see Jak El-Hai, *The Lobotomist: A Maverick Medical Genius and His Tragic Quest to Rid the World of Mental Illness* (Hoboken, NJ: Wiley, 2007).

22. For an account of Dr. Freeman's work at Athens, with an account by Dr. Wolfard Baumgaertel of Freeman's third visit to Athens in 1954, see Cordingley, *Stories of Medicine,* 50–52.

23. Hubert Haymond Fockler, hospital memo dated December 13, 1956, Athens State Hospital Superintendents' Correspondence. Dr. Harry Chovnick (superintendent at Athens, 1967–73) doubted Freeman's lobotomy outcome research and speculated that lobotomized patients were getting better anyway. Cordingley, *Stories of Medicine,* 302.

24. Athens State Hospital, *Annual Report of the Athens State Hospital for the Fiscal Year Ending June 30, 1953,* 9. Mahn Center for Archives and Special Collections, Ohio University Libraries. The Red Cross Gray Lady Service began in 1918 at Walter Reed Army Hospital; the Gray Ladies were so named because of their uniform of gray dresses and veils. The function of the service was to provide friendly personal service such as recreational and educational activities for patients in hospitals, clinics, and other institutions. Fifty thousand Gray Ladies served during World War II. Sixty-three women volunteered as Gray Ladies at the Athens asylum during the 1950s. In the 1960s, the Gray Lady Service was folded into the Red Cross Volunteer Services. Katherine Ziff, "The Gray Ladies: Social Capital and Community at the Athens Asylum for the Insane," presentation at the Fourth Annual Conference of the Women of Appalachia, Zanesville, Ohio, October 25, 2002.

25. *Fiscal Year 1952–1953 Annual Report of the Athens State Hospital to the Ohio Division of Mental Hygiene, Department of Public Welfare, July 1, 1953,* 4. Mahn Center for Archives and Special Collections, Ohio University Libraries.

26. Ibid., 11.

27. Psychologist Catherine Semans reported on the administration to patients of tests to assess cognitive ability, such as the Wechsler and the Stanford-Binet; personality structure and psychopathology, such as the Minnesota Multiphasic Personality Inventory (MMPI); neurological function, such as the Bender-Gestalt; projective tests, such as the Rorschach and Draw-a-Person; and career interest inventories, such as the Kuder Preference Test. In 1953, asylum psychologists had twenty-five tests on hand for patients; 311 tests were administered to 151 patients that year. Athens State Hospital, 1953 annual report.

28. Wes Lindamood, "Thorazine," *Chemical and Engineering News* 83 (2005): 5.

29. Grob, *Mad among Us,* 271–73.

30. Mrs. Szot was an attendant and then a nurse at Danvers State Hospital during the 1950s and 1960s. She described the grim laundry situation during outbreaks of illness: "With so many people crowded in, it was not surprising when small epidemics broke out. There would be dozens of diarrhea cases at one time. The patients would be brought several at a time into the showers and literally hosed down to clean the filth. It didn't hurt them physically in any way. Some of them were dying from dehydration caused by diarrhea. All the clothes were soiled at one point, so most of the patients had nothing to wear. I remember telling my husband there wasn't a patient on the floor who had a stitch of clothes on. Danvers had its own laundry room complete with staff or washing bedsheets and patients' clothes. Sometimes a diarrhea epidemic would create such a pile of rancid, filthy clothes and sheets that it would take the crew several days of bleaching and disinfecting to get back to normal." Angelina Szot and Barbara Stilwell, *Danvers State: Memoirs of a Nurse in the Asylum* (Bloomington, IN: Authorhouse, 2004), 86–87.

31. Quoted in Cordingley, *Stories of Medicine,* 298.

32. David Malawista (clinical and forensic psychologist, former director of psychology at Athens Mental Health Center), discussion with the author, July 2010.

33. Marilyn Sue Foster (superintendent at Athens Mental Health Center, 1977–85), discussion with the author, July 2010. Dr. Foster, a social psychologist, began her career at the Athens Mental Health Center in 1966 as a researcher. She was given an office in Cottage O (a ward for men) and a desk. The patients of Cottage O helped her find things to furnish the rest of her work space. Among Dr. Foster's many accomplishments as assistant superintendent and then superintendent was securing Medicare approval for the mental health center.

34. William Stanley "Billy" Milligan, the first person in the United States to be found not guilty of a major crime by reason of insanity with a diagnosis of multiple personality disorder, was a patient at the asylum at Athens. For more information on his life and his stay at the asylum, see Daniel Keyes, *The Minds of Billy Milligan* (New York: Bantam Books, 1982).

35. Malawista to author, July 2010.

36. Sally Walters, "History of Center Goes on Sale Saturday," *Athens (OH) Messenger,* December 2, 1977.

37. Christopher Payne, *Asylum: Inside the Closed World of State Mental Hospitals* (Cambridge, MA: MIT Press, 2009).

38. http://www.kirkbridebuildings.com/.

39. NBBJ, *Architectural Master Plan: Ohio University, The Ridges* (Columbus, OH: NBBJ, 2001), 66.

40. See http://www.dairybarn.org.

41. For details, see http://www.ohio.edu/avionics/radarhill/index.cfm.

42. "Ridges Plan Critics Given the Floor," *Athens (OH) Messenger,* October 1, 1992.

43. Pam Callahan (Ohio University architect, retired), discussion with the author, November 5, 2010.

44. Ohio University, *Vision Ohio: Ohio University Master Planning Report* (Athens: Ohio University, November 2006), 89.

45. BOHM-NBBJ, *Ohio University Comprehensive Land Use Study: The Ridges* (Columbus, OH: BOHM-NBBJ, 1989), 111.

46. Ridges Cemeteries Committee, *Visitor's Guide: The State Psychiatric Hospital Cemeteries and The Ridges Cemeteries Nature Walk* (Athens: Ohio University Printing and Graphic Services).

BIBLIOGRAPHY

Abbott, John S. C., and Russell H. Conwell. *Lives of the Presidents of the United States of America: From Washington to the Present Time.* Portland, ME: H. Hallett, 1882.

Abrams, Eliot, and AnnCorinne Freter, eds. *The Emergence of the Moundbuilders: The Archaeology of Tribal Societies in Southeastern Ohio.* Athens: Ohio University Press, 2005.

Alderman, Derek H. "Integrating Space into a Reactive Theory of the Asylum: Evidence from Post–Civil War Georgia." *Health and Place* 3 (1997): 111–22.

Athens Journal. "Athens County Roads Are Now Three Feet Deep in Mud," February 2, 1893.

Athens Mental Health Center Patient Records. Athens Lunatic Asylum Manuscript Collection (MS #263). Mahn Center for Archives and Special Collections, Ohio University Libraries. Cited in notes as AMHC Patient Records.

Athens (OH) Messenger. "Death of George Link, Landscape Gardener at Hospital for Thirty-Two Years," August 16, 1903.

———. "Grounds of State Hospital Most Beautiful of Middle West," May 3, 1955.

———. "History of Athens Mental Health Center: Hospital-Community Relationship Spans 121 Years," March 21, 1988.

———. "Laying the Cornerstone of the New Asylum: Vast Concourses of People." November 12, 1868.

———. Local Matters, January 29 and May 27, 1880.

———. "Ridges Plan Critics Given the Floor," October 1, 1992.

———. "Samuel Whitely, A Tramp." January 8, 1880.

Athens State Hospital. *Annual Report for the Year Ending November 15, 1913.* Mahn Center for Archives and Special Collections, Ohio University Libraries.

———. *Annual Report of the Athens State Hospital for the Fiscal Year Ending June 30, 1953.* Mahn Center for Archives and Special Collections, Ohio University Libraries.

———. *Case Book for Female Patients 1–167,* 1874. State Archives Series 141. Ohio Historical Society Archives/Library.

———. *Case Book for Male Patients 1–179,* 1874. State Archives Series 141. Ohio Historical Society Archives/Library.

———. *Fiscal Year 1952–1953 Annual Report of the Athens State Hospital to the Ohio Division of Mental Hygiene, Department of Public Welfare, July 1, 1953.*

———. *Thirty-Eighth Report of the Athens State Hospital for the Year Ending November 15, 1913 to the Ohio Board of Administration.* Athens, OH: n.p., 1913.

Athens State Hospital Superintendents' Correspondence. Athens Lunatic Asylum Manuscript Collection (MS #263). Mahn Center for Archives and Special Collections, Ohio University Libraries. Cited in the notes as Athens State Hospital Superintendents' Correspondence.

Ballard Manuscript Collection (MS #23). Mahn Center for Archives and Special Collections, Ohio University Libraries.

Bateman, J. Fremont, and H. Warren Dunham. "The State Mental Hospital as a Specialized Community Experience." *American Journal of Psychiatry* 105 (1948): 445–48.

Berry, John H. "Historical Sketch No. 17: The Athens State Hospital, . . . 1929." Report prepared for the Ohio Department of Public Welfare. Vertical files for the Athens Mental Health Center in Mahn Center for Archives and Special Collections, Ohio University Libraries.

Blankenbeker, Steven D. "The Paving Brick Industry in Ohio." *Ohio Geology* 3 (1999): 1–2.

Board of State Charities. *Ohio Executive Documents: Annual Reports for 1879–1881.* Columbus, OH: Nevins and Myers, 1880, 1881; G. J. Brand and Co., 1882.

Board of Trustees of the Athens Asylum for the Insane. *Ohio Executive Documents: Annual Reports for 1878–1893.* Columbus, OH: Nevins and Myers, 1879–81; G. J. Brand and Co., 1882–84; Westbote Co., 1885–92; Laning Printing Co., 1893–94.

Board of Trustees of the Athens Hospital for the Insane. *Ohio Executive Documents: Annual Reports for 1876, 1877.* Columbus, OH: Nevins and Myers, 1877–78.

Board of Trustees of the Athens Lunatic Asylum. *Ohio Executive Documents: Annual Reports for 1871.* Columbus, OH: Nevins and Myers, 1872.

———. *Ohio Executive Documents: Annual Reports for 1872.* Columbus, OH: Nevins and Myers, 1873.

BOHM-NBBJ. *Ohio University Comprehensive Land Use Study: The Ridges.* Columbus, OH: BOHM-NBBJ, 1989.

Broder, Sherri. *Tramps, Unfit Mothers and Neglected Children: Negotiating the Family in Late Nineteenth-Century Philadelphia.* Philadelphia: University of Pennsylvania Press, 2002.

Cerney, Charles I. *The Chronicles of Medicine in Muskingum County, Ohio, 1800–2000.* Zanesville, OH: privately published.

Connett, Lucinda Pickett, Collection. Athens County (Ohio) Museum and Historical Society.

Conwell, Russell H. *Life and Service of Governor Rutherford B. Hayes.* Boston: Franklin Press, 1876.

Cordingley, Gary E. *Stories of Medicine in Athens County, Ohio.* Baltimore, MD: Gateway Press, 2006.

Daniel, Robert L. *Athens, Ohio: The Village Years.* Athens: Ohio University Press, 1997.

Dean, Eric. *Shook Over Hell: Post-traumatic Stress, Vietnam, and the Civil War.* Cambridge, MA: Harvard University Press, 1997.

Edelstein, Emma J., and Ludwig Edelstein. *Asclepius: Collection and Interpretation of the Testimonies.* Baltimore, MD: Johns Hopkins University Press, 1945.

El-Hai, Jak. *The Lobotomist: A Maverick Medical Genius and His Tragic Quest to Rid the World of Mental Illness.* Hoboken, NJ: Wiley, 2007.

Eyman, Henry C. "Massillon State Hospital." In *The Institutional Care of the Insane in the United States and Canada,* edited by Henry Mills Hurd et al., 3:330–32. Baltimore, MD: Johns Hopkins University Press, 1916. Available online at books.google.com.

Faust, Drew Gilpin. *This Republic of Suffering: Death and the American Civil War.* New York: Alfred A. Knopf, 2008.

Floyd, Barbara, Kimberly Brownlee, Tamara Jones, Jennifer Free, and David Chelminski. *From Institutions to Independence: A History of People with Disabilities in Northwest Ohio—An Exhibition.* Toledo: Ward M. Canaday Center for Special Collections, University Libraries, University of Toledo, 2009.

Foucault, Michel. *Madness and Civilization.* New York: Random House, 1965.

Frost, Robert. *The Poetry of Robert Frost.* New York: Henry Holt and Co., 1969.

Gerlach-Spriggs, Nancy, Richard Enoch Kaufman, and Sam Bass Warner Jr. *Restorative Gardens: The Healing Landscape.* New Haven, CT: Yale University Press, 1998.

Gollaher, David. *Voice for the Mad: The Life of Dorothea Dix.* New York: Free Press, 1995.

Grob, Gerald N. *The Mad among Us: A History of the Care of America's Mentally Ill.* New York: Free Press, 1994.

———. "The Transformation of the Mental Hospital in the United States." *American Behavioral Scientist* 28 (1985): 639–54.

"Haerlin, Herman (Chief Gardener at National Military Home)." *Gardening* 14 (January 1, 1906): 354.

Haerlin, Herman. "Report of Commissioner Haerlin." In *Annual Report of the Ohio State Board of Agriculture for 1888,* 58–59. Columbus, OH: Westbote Co., 1881.

Hagdorn, Ann. *Beyond the River: The Untold Story of the Heroes of the Underground Railroad*. New York: Simon and Schuster, 2002.

Halstead, Murat. *Life and Distinguished Services of Hon. William McKinley and the Great Issues of 1896*. Philadelphia: Edgewood Publishing Co., 1896.

Hannibal, J.T., and R.A. Davis. "The Cleves Tunnel, a Rare Extant Example of the Use of Buena Vista Stone for a Canal Structure near Cincinnati, Ohio." In *Proceedings of the 40th Forum on the Geology of Industrial Minerals, May 2–7, 2004*, edited by N. R. Shafer and D. A. DeChurch, 64–69. Bloomington: Indiana Geological Survey Occasional Paper 67, 2004.

Haworth, Paul Leland. *The Hayes-Tilden Disputed Presidential Election of 1876*. Cleveland: Burrows, 1906.

Hayes, Rutherford B. "Annual Message to the General Assembly." In *Ohio Executive Documents: Annual Reports for 1869*. Columbus, OH: Columbus Printing Company, 1870.

———. "Annual Message to the General Assembly." In *Ohio Executive Documents: Annual Reports for 1870*. Columbus, OH: Nevins and Myers, 1871.

———. *The Diary and Letters of Rutherford B. Hayes, Nineteenth President of the United States*. Edited by Charles Richard Williams. Columbus: Ohio State Archeological and Historical Society, 1922.

Hayes, Samuel P. *The Response to Industrialism*. Chicago: University of Chicago Press, 1995.

History of Cleveland and Its Environs, A. Chicago: Lewis Publishing, 1918.

Holden, William H. "Sixth Annual Report of the Athens Asylum for the Insane." In *Ohio Executive Documents: Annual Reports for 1879*. Columbus, OH: Nevins and Myers, 1880.

Hoover, Thomas. *The History of Ohio University*. Athens: Ohio University Press, 1954.

Johnson, William Parker, Letters. Manuscript Collection #173. Mahn Center for Archives and Special Collections, Ohio University Libraries. Cited in notes as Johnson Letters.

Keyes, Daniel. *The Minds of Billy Milligan*. New York: Bantam Books, 1982.

Kirkbride, Thomas S. *On the Construction, Organization and General Arrangements of Hospitals for the Insane, with Some Remarks on Insanity and Its Treatment*. Philadelphia: Pennsylvania Hospital for the Insane, 1854.

———. *On the Construction, Organization and General Arrangements of Hospitals for the Insane*. 2nd ed. 1880; repr., New York: Arno Press, 1973.

Knepper, George. *Ohio and Its People*. Kent, OH: Kent State University, 1989.

Lake, D. J. *Atlas of Athens County, Ohio*. Philadelphia: Titus, Simmons and Titus, 1875.

Lindamood, Wes. "Thorazine." *Chemical and Engineering News* 83 (2005).

Marinski, Deborah. "Unfortunate Minds: Mental Insanity in Ohio, 1883–1909." PhD diss., University of Toledo, 2006.

Marlow, David. *Psychological and Psychosocial Consequences of Combat and Deployment*. Washington, DC: National Defense Research Institute, 2001.

Mitchell, S. Weir. "Address before the Fiftieth Annual Meeting of the American Medico-Psychological Association, Philadelphia, May 16, 1894." *American Journal of Psychiatry* 151 (1994): 28–36. Reprinted from the *Journal of Nervous and Mental Disease*, July 1894.

Morris, S. Brent. *Cornerstones of Freemasonry: A Masonic Tradition*. Washington, DC: Masonic Supreme Council, 1993.

Murphy, James. *An Archeological History of the Hocking Valley*. Athens: Ohio University Press, 1989.

NBBJ. *Architectural Master Plan: Ohio University, The Ridges*. Columbus, OH: NBBJ, 2001.

New People's Universal Cyclopedia of Universal Knowledge, The. New York: Phillips and Hunt, 1885.

Norbury, Frank B. "Dorothea Dix and the Founding of Illinois' First Mental Hospital." *Journal of the Illinois State Historical Society* 92 (1999): 13–29.

Noyes, Edward F. "Annual Message to the General Assembly." In *Ohio Executive Documents: Annual Reports for 1873*. Columbus, OH: Nevin and Myers, 1874.

O'Bleness Family Collection. Manuscript Collection #151. Mahn Center for Archives and Special Collections, Ohio University Libraries.

Ohio University. *Vision Ohio: Ohio University Master Planning Report.* Athens: Ohio University, November 2006.

Paulson, George W., and Marion E. Sherman. *Hilltop: A Hospital and a Sanctuary for Healing; Its Past and Its Future.* Fremont, OH: Lesher, 2008.

Payne, Christopher. *Asylum: Inside the Closed World of State Mental Hospitals.* Cambridge, MA: MIT Press, 2009.

Perry, James. *Touched with Fire: Five Presidents and the Civil War Battles That Made Them.* New York: Public Affairs, 2003.

Phillips, Hazel, and Lawrence Gray. *Governors of Ohio.* Columbus: Ohio Historical Society, 1952.

Picturesque Athens Asylum: Views In and About Athens Asylum for the Insane. Columbus: Baker Photogravure Co., 1893.

Pinel, Philippe. *Traité médico-philosophique sur l'aliénation mentale.* Translated by D. D. Davis. Birmingham, AL: Classics of Medicine Library, 1983.

Porter, Roy. *Madness: A Brief History.* Oxford: Oxford University Press, 2002.

Progressive Men of Northern Ohio. Cleveland: Plain Dealer Publishing Co., 1906.

Putnam, Robert. *Bowling Alone: The Collapse and Revival of American Community.* New York: Simon and Schuster, 2001.

Ricord, P. *A Practical Treatise on Venereal Diseases.* New York: Gordon, 1842.

Ridges Cemeteries Committee. *Visitor's Guide: The State Psychiatric Hospital Cemeteries and The Ridges Cemeteries Nature Walk.* Athens: Ohio University Printing and Graphic Services.

Roberts, F. David. *The Social Conscience of the Early Victorians.* Stanford: Stanford University Press, 2002.

Rybczynski, Witold. *A Clearing in the Distance: Frederick Law Olmsted and America in the Nineteenth Century.* New York: Scribner, 1999.

Scott, W. H. "Memorial for Alonzo B. Richardson." In *Proceedings of the American Medico-Psychological Association at the Sixtieth Annual Meeting.* St. Louis: American Psychological Association, 1904.

Scull, Andrew. *The Insanity of Place/The Place of Insanity: Essays on the History of Psychiatry.* New York: Routledge, 2006.

———. "Psychiatry and Social Control in the Nineteenth and Twentieth Centuries." *History of Psychiatry* 2 (1991): 149–69.

———. "A Quarter Century of the History of Psychiatry." *Journal of the History of the Behavioral Sciences* 35 (1999): 239–46.

———. *Social Order/Mental Disorder: Anglo-American Psychiatry in Historical Perspective.* Berkeley: University of California Press, 1989.

Sitton, Sarah C. *Life at the Texas State Lunatic Asylum, 1857–1997.* College Station: Texas A&M University Press, 1999.

Smyth, Fiona. "Medical Geography: Therapeutic Places, Spaces and Networks." *Progress in Human Geography* 29 (2005): 488–95.

Sternberg, Esther M. *Healing Spaces: The Science of Place and Well-Being.* Cambridge, MA: Belknap Press, 2009.

Szot, Angelina, and Barbara Stilwell. *Danvers State: Memoirs of a Nurse in the Asylum.* Bloomington, IN: Authorhouse, 2004.

Theriot, Nancy. "Diagnosing Unnatural Motherhood: Nineteenth Century Physicians and Puerperal Insanity." In *Women and Health in America: Historical Readings,* edited by Judith Walzer Leavitt, 403–17. Madison: University of Wisconsin Press, 1999.

Tipton, S. C. *Athens County Illustrated Progress of One Hundred Years Centennial.* Athens, OH: Messenger and Herald, 1897.

Tom, Fred Lee. *Topographic Map of Ohio University and Vicinity.* Hand-drawn map, 1911. Collection of the Mahn Center for Archives and Special Collections, Ohio University Libraries.

Tomes, Nancy. *The Art of Asylum-Keeping: Thomas Story Kirkbride and the Origins of American Psychiatry*. Philadelphia: University of Pennsylvania Press, 1984.

Waite, Diana S. "History of Construction of the Athens State Hospital." In *Master Plan for Kennedy Museum: Feasibility Study*, 3–17. Albany: John G. Waite Associates, 1999.

Walters, Sally. "History of Center Goes on Sale Saturday." *Athens (OH) Messenger*, December 2, 1977.

Wotton, Henry. *The Elements of Architecture by Sir Henry Wotton, a Facsimili Reprint of the First Edition (London, 1624)*. Edited by Frederick Hard. Charlottesville: University Press of Virginia, 1968.

Young, Thomas L. "Inaugural Message." In *Ohio Executive Documents: Annual Reports for 1876*. Columbus, OH: Nevins and Myers, 1877.

Zenner, Dr. Phillip. Manuscript Collection (MS #44). Mahn Center for Archives and Special Collections, Ohio University Libraries.

Zanesville (OH) Signal, 1925. Photograph edited and provided by Dr. Charles I. Cerney, Zanesville, Ohio.

Ziff, Katherine. "Asylum and Community: Connections between the Athens Lunatic Asylum and the Village of Athens, 1867–1893." PhD diss., Ohio University, 2004.

———. "The Gray Ladies: Social Capital and Community at the Athens Asylum for the Insane." Presentation at the Fourth Annual Conference of the Women of Appalachia, Zanesville, Ohio, October 25, 2002.

Ziff, Katherine, David Thomas, and Patricia Beamish. "Asylum and Community: The Athens Lunatic Asylum in Nineteenth-Century Ohio." *History of Psychiatry* 19 (2008): 409–32.

Zimmerman, Carolyn, Ünige Laskay, and Glen P. Jackson. "Analysis of Suspected Trace Human Remains from an Indoor Concrete Surface." *Journal of Forensic Sciences* 6 (2008): 1437–42.

Index

Buena Vista freestone, 63, 200n1
Buffalo State Hospital, 126
Buxton, William, 146

Calkins, W. R., 205n7
Campbell, James E., 110, 122
Cantino, Phillip D., 189
caregivers, 125–64
Carthage, OH, 113
casebooks, 14, 26, 28, 35, 43, 142; men, 31, 33, 44, 49;
    women, 34, 50, 51, 62, 142, 151
Caul, David, 185
cemetery, 43, 151, 198n44
Central Ohio Lunatic Asylum (Central Asylum,
    Columbus State Hospital, Hilltop), 2, 71, 79, 107,
    112, 114, 120, 161, 167; fire, 14, 69, 70; history of,
    193n2; patients from, 14, 32, 34, 41, 47
Champlin, Verda, 172
chapel, 73, 78, 79
child bearing, 36
childbirth, 27, 34, 35, 150, 197n25
children, 4, 15, 32, 36, 47, 51, 52, 57–59, 61, 66, 130, 150,
    155, 159, 192
Children's Garden, 184
Chillicothe, OH, 32, 33, 47, 127, 163
Chovnick, Harry, 182, 207n23
Christmas, 152, 153
C. H. Warden & Brothers, 205n7
Cincinnati, OH, 2, 198n47, 199n59; brothel, 17;
    contractors, 64; Gundry, Richard, 112; Haerlin,
    Herman, 106, 125, 126, 127; Hayes, Rutherford
    B., 112; Longview Asylum, 107, 113; patients, 162,
    197n19; police, 17; Richardson, A. B., 161; Rutter,
    Henly, 114; Southern Asylum at, 20, 29, 199n57
Civilian Conservation Corps, 191
Civil War, x, 1, 2, 19, 20, 40, 66, 71, 105, 159, 195n40;
    Antietam, battle of, 9; Atlanta, battle of,
    40, 71, 197n24, 205n18; cannonading, 30, 40;
    Chickamauga, battle of, 40, 71, 197n24,, 205n18;
    Confederates, 19; Corinth, battle of, 40, 197n24;
    post-traumatic stress, 19; Shiloh, battle of, 40;
    veteran, 19, 35, 40, 41, 49, 195n40; weaponry, 19
Clark, Sarah M., 147
Clarke, P. H., 22, 109, 117, 118, 119, 139, 141;
    complaints about behavior of, 114–17
Cleveland, OH, 2, 29, 70, 71, 107, 112
coal, 13, 17, 78, 108, 110, 113, 154, 205n7; miners, 17,
    195n32; wheelers, 77, 154
Coates, Mrs. William, 153
Coates farm, 185
cocaine, 50
Columbian Medical School (Georgetown Medical
    School), 123
Columbus, OH, 1, 2, 24, 28, 29, 106, 159, 198n47;
    Centennial Fair of 1888, 127; Dorothea Dix, 107;
    sanatorium, 167. See also Central Ohio Lunatic
    Asylum (Central Asylum, Columbus State
    Hospital, Hilltop)
combat fatigue, 19

commitment, 36, 37, 40, 41, 48, 52, 55, 196n2, 199n56,
    200n68; decisions, 61, 151; documents and papers,
    14, 27, 30, 34, 35, 47, 55, 57, 58, 59, 61, 196n2;
    hearings, 25, 48
Community Mental Health Act of 1963, 181, 182
concerts, 144, 160, 161
Connett, George, 156
Connett, Lucinda Pickett, 154–56
conservatory, 22, 121, 140
contracts, 67, 107, 108, 110, 154
cornerstone, 7, 68, 194n10
Cosmos Club, 123
Cottage B, 177
Cottage L, 189
Cottage M, 187
Cottage O, 169, 208n33
cottage plan, 122, 164–67, 169, 190
Cottage R, 169
Cox, Charlotte, 180
Cox, Jacob D., 71, 111
Creed, Charles Harry, Jr., 180, 181
Creed, Charles Harry, Jr., Mrs., 180
Crosby, Bing, 181
Crumbacker, W. P., 122

dairy, 108, 136, 153, 158, 159, 177, 181, 188
Dairy Barn Arts Center, 188, 190
Danvers State Hospital, 182, 207n30
Davies, John M., 68
Davis & Son, 205n7
Day, D. W. H., 63, 65
Dayton, OH, 2, 29, 58, 68, 107, 112, 119, 162, 199n57
deinstitutionalization, 167, 181, 183
dementia, 27, 30, 32, 47, 50, 57, 151, 166, 175, 197n11
depression, 4, 27, 30, 32, 35, 47, 106, 197n11
Devlyn, Anna, 171, 172
dining rooms: employee, 75; officers, 72; patients, 23,
    67, 78, 122, 144, 146, 148; wards, 74, 77, 78
Dix, Dorothea, 107, 123
Dixmont State Hospital, 8
drugs, 153, 179; morphine, 35, 37, 39. See also
    medications
Dunlap, C. O., 109
dynamometer, 31, 197n14
D. Zenner & Sons, 202n27, 205n7

Earle, Pliny, 206n5
Eastern Lunatic Asylum, 167
Eckle, Catherine, 130
electric cabinet treatment, 176
electric lights, 78, 117, 147, 152
electric shock therapy (electroconvulsive therapy),
    178–80
epilepsy, 25, 26, 30, 37, 58, 114, 196n2, n4, 199n57
exercise, 8, 126, 132, 136, 138, 139, 144, 204n29
Eyman, Henry C., 202n46

Farrer, Nancy, 112
Fergus Falls asylum, 187